I Think My Child Needs Braces... Answers To The Most
Common Questions Parents Have About Orthodontics
© 2018 Dr. Ryan Tamburrino / Burleson Media Group

ISBN: 978-1-970095-02-9

TABLE OF CONTENTS

FOREWORD
Why Read This Book?

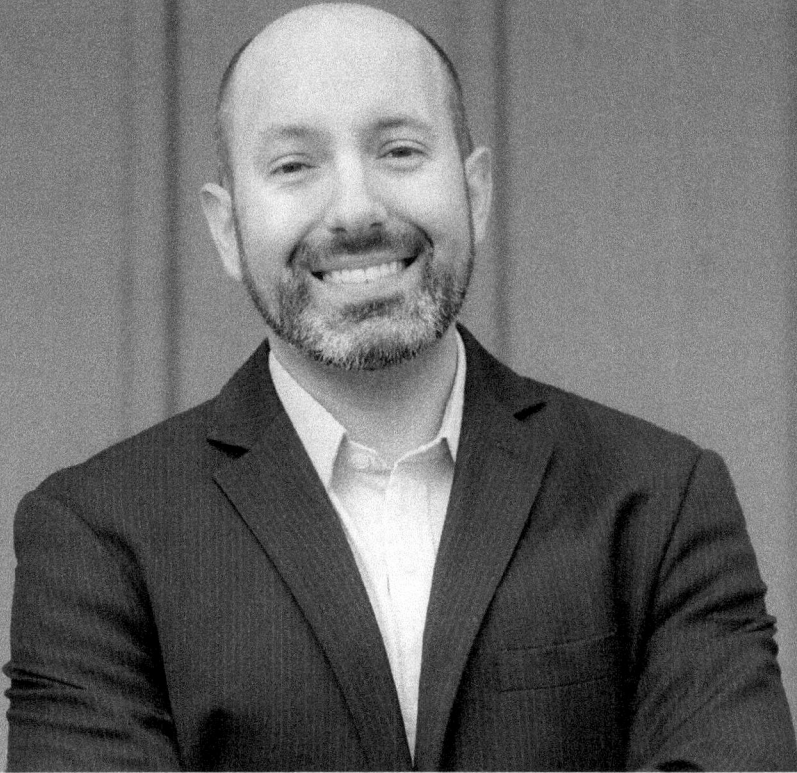

Hi there! My name is Dr. Ryan Tamburrino. You can read all about me on the back cover (and I think that's more than enough of this book's real estate dedicated to me). As an orthodontist, I could talk all day and devote volumes of text to my love for teeth and reasons for wanting to create amazing smiles! However, that's not why you sat down to read this book. You didn't open the cover to learn about me or any of my passions. You opened this book to learn about orthodontic treatment and how to make a good decision for your family.

Therefore, this book is not a celebration of me. It is solely dedicated to help YOU, both with understanding the braces process, and giving YOU solid, unbiased information to make YOU a better informed parent. The goals are twofold: 1. help you understand when and why you should seek care from an orthodontist, and 2. how to help you choose the best doctor to provide the care.

Most people have heard things about the orthodontic profession and know a little about how it works. At the very least, most people know that they are seeking orthodontic care because they want straight teeth and a great smile. They also realize they will need to wear some type of appliance to get it, whether that be braces, clear aligners, or any number of other options available.

There's an abundance of information (and even mis-information!) about braces and orthodontics out there. However, even with this knowledge being readily available, most families I speak to are still pretty confused when it comes to knowing when they should see an orthodontist, how to choose the best orthodontic provider for their family, and understanding how the orthodontic process works.

I believe an orthodontic journey for a family should be about more than just teeth, which is something that seems to be forgotten in today's hectic, aesthetic-forward society. Orthodontics is about creating a healthy, functional bite to last for the rest of your life. It's about teamwork, forming trust, and fostering mutual respect among your family, your orthodontist, and the office team. It's about realizing there's a living, breathing unique human attached to those 28 pearly whites. It's about giving your child's confidence room to grow and letting their personality shine!

Having been in practice for over a decade and having the privilege of working with hundreds and hundreds of amazing families, I've heard several questions get repeated over and over in consult after consult. To me, their constant resurfacing means they are real concerns, and, more importantly, these questions are not being answered satisfactorily from speaking with family/friends, or with personal research conducted on the internet.

I often find that people are genuinely confused when they come to see me for the first time, so the purpose of this book is to help provide clarity and education. When you're done reading, things should be crystal clear in your mind for what to do next for your child, if anything at all! (Not to mention you'll also get massive bragging rights with your friends when you can answer these questions confidently for them!)

I've listed below the 10 most common questions that families ask me during their initial visit. See how many you already know the answers to:

1. Why should I even see an orthodontist?
2. How can I tell the difference among orthodontic providers?
3. What's the difference between an orthodontist and my family dentist?

4. What will the braces experience be like?
5. What are treatment options that I have other than braces?
6. When is the best time to get started?
7. How does my dental insurance work?
8. How can I make orthodontic care fit into my family's budget?
9. Does my child need adult teeth removed?
10. What happens when the braces come off?

If you scored 100%, you can put this book down now - you're either a trained orthodontist already, cheated and read the rest of the book first, or you have super mental Jedi powers!

If you're hesitant or don't know the answers to any of them, then this book is exactly the help you need. Grab a coffee or other beverage of choice and continue reading! I promise – there's minimal technical/medical jargon or mumbo jumbo so it's an easy read, but it's one that's packed with honest information!

Throughout this book, I'll go into detail for each of the above questions, as well as give you some bonus material at the end. When you're finished, you'll have enough solid information to embark on your child's smile journey as a well-informed, confident parent.

With the basics now out of the way, you can just focus your energy on the important questions to ask yourself...such as, is this orthodontist I'm visiting someone I can trust, and, if so, when can I get started!

Happy smiles to you, and all the best on your journey!

Ryan K. Tamburrino, DMD

Co-Founder – Center for Orthodontic Excellence
International Orthodontic Educator – Complete Clinical Orthodontics System
Former Faculty – University of Pennsylvania School of Dental Medicine,
Department of Orthodontics
Author – Orthodontic Treatment Design (Textbook) & numerous clinical publications
Husband to an amazing wife and dad to 2 incredible boys.

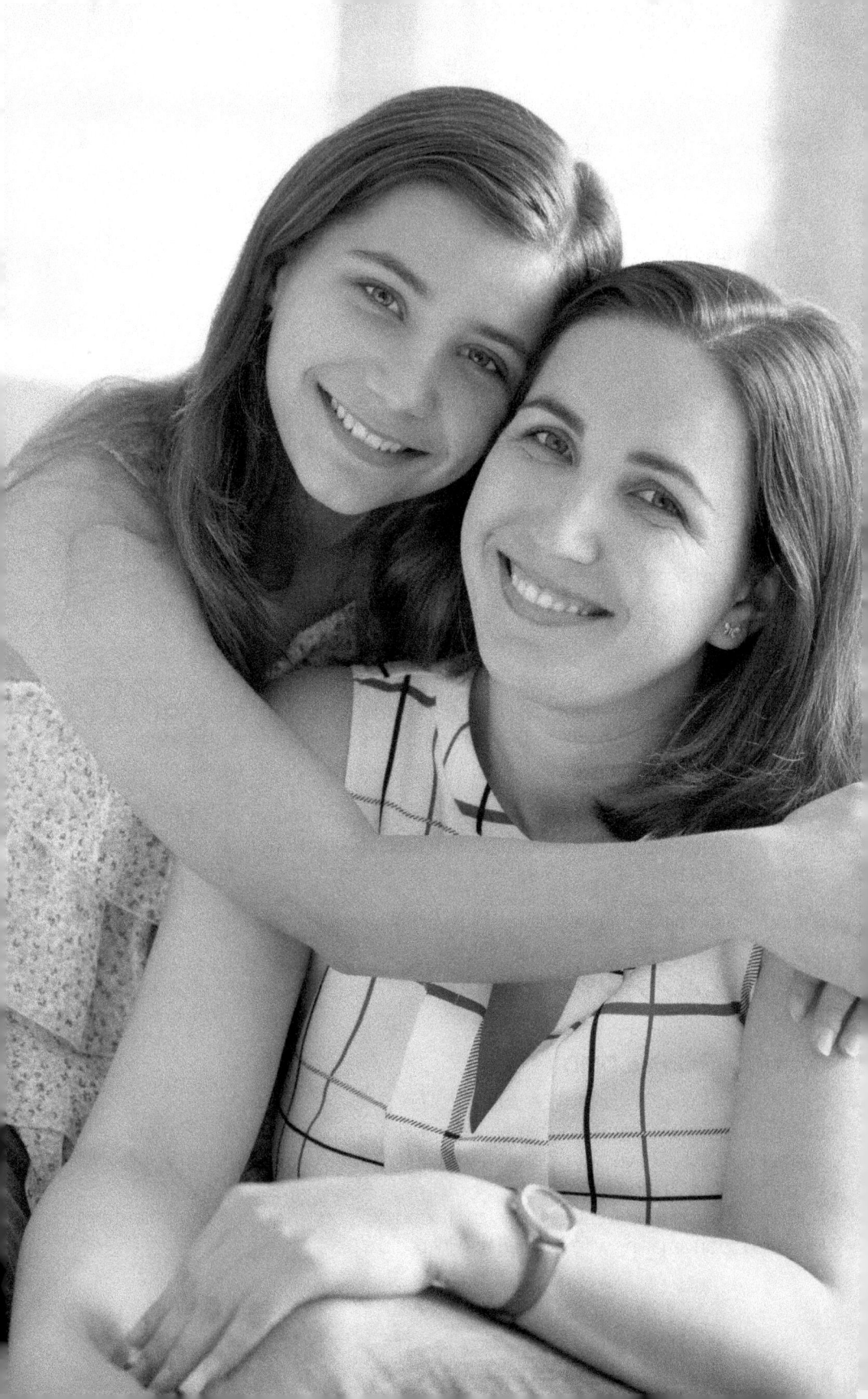

INTRODUCTION

I know this is what you probably thinking, so I just want to put it out there before we even start...

> *Hey Dr. T, I remember when I had braces or my friends had braces when we were growing up. It was miserable and we looked like complete dorks! Is that still the case?*

Well, for one, it's not 1970 or 1980 anymore. While some fashion and music trends from those eras are still en vogue, not much about orthodontics still is. The days of painful adjustments, frequent visits, and long appointments are over. Today's orthodontic technology is comfortable, often allows for extended intervals between office visits, and provides for quick appointments that easily fit into your day.

Secondly, the aesthetics have dramatically changed for the better. Gone is the stigma of being called "metal mouth" and cartoon images of kids in braces being made fun of. Gone are the miles of wire tying everything together. Gone are the severe speech and eating issues. Modern appliances for orthodontics blend nicely into the teeth (and there are also invisible options available!) Orthodontics is not "geeky" and is well accepted as a "normal" part of growing up. Actually, most kids are pretty excited to get going and think it's "cool" to have braces!

Third, orthodontics has also become more affordable than ever. With many practitioners offering extended financing options, accepting flexible spending account monies, utilizing employer provided dental benefits, and customizing payment plans, the rigid payment structures are a thing of the past. There is now no reason to ever turn a dental problem into a financial problem. Affordable options abound!

Now that those three misconceptions are out of the way, you can take a deep breath. Braces won't be incredibly painful. You won't have your life inconvenienced. Your child won't look ridiculous. You won't have to choose between going on vacation or getting a great smile for your kid. It's all going to be ok...I promise!

So let's jump right in...

CHAPTER 1

Why is My Child's Smile So Important?

Orthodontics is about more than getting braces just for the sake of getting braces or correcting crooked, spaced, or funky-looking teeth. One's smile is the gateway to their personality! In addition:

1. Both kids and adults with great smiles feel better about themselves, and that can greatly increase their self-confidence, reduce teasing, and improve social well-being.

2. Straight teeth function better, are easier to clean, and are more likely to last a lifetime. That saves a whole lot of time, future dental expenses, and discomfort as your child matures into an adult.

3. People with straight, well-aligned teeth can avoid gum disease, which has been linked to heart disease and other serious health issues.

4. A properly functioning bite lowers the risk of temporomandibular joint disorders (TMJ pain) and chronic headaches.

5. While not directly affected by just aligning teeth, orthodontists know the importance of breathing well and getting good sleep have on a child's development. They have the tools and knowledge to address a potential breathing problem before it becomes more serious.

6. Eating becomes a ton easier and more enjoyable when all the teeth work together properly

While it does seem like braces are a "rite of passage" for kids, many people can eat, speak, and breathe just fine with a less than perfect bite (and I've seen some pretty wild ones in my day!) However, with the personal confidence that comes with a gorgeous, bright smile and straight teeth, many parents are electing to pursue orthodontic treatment for their kids (and also themselves!)

While the obvious benefits of orthodontic treatment are easily seen with a great smile, there is much more benefit to the going through the process beyond just getting straight teeth! Orthodontists are the experts of the whole chewing system, and we are trained to know how to get the teeth, jaws, and chewing muscles to work together harmoniously.

Orthodontists also know the importance of breathing and it's effects on poor sleep, sleep apnea, and the growth potential of your child's body and brain. This stuff is not directly affected by simply aligning teeth, but we have the tools and resources to help address a potential problem before it actually becomes a problem! Fortunately, it's not the case or an issue for many children, but it's nice to know that someone is looking out!

So yeah, a great smile with straight teeth is, at the very baseline, what orthodontists will give your child! However, many not so obvious reasons for orthodontic treatment, including preventing future dental and developmental issues before they become severe, are also hallmarks of an orthodontist's care.   There will be much more on these topics later. For now, though, let's start with the big question on your mind...

> **Call us at 484.730.1921 or go to www.coesmiles.com to schedule your own Customized Smile Analysis.**

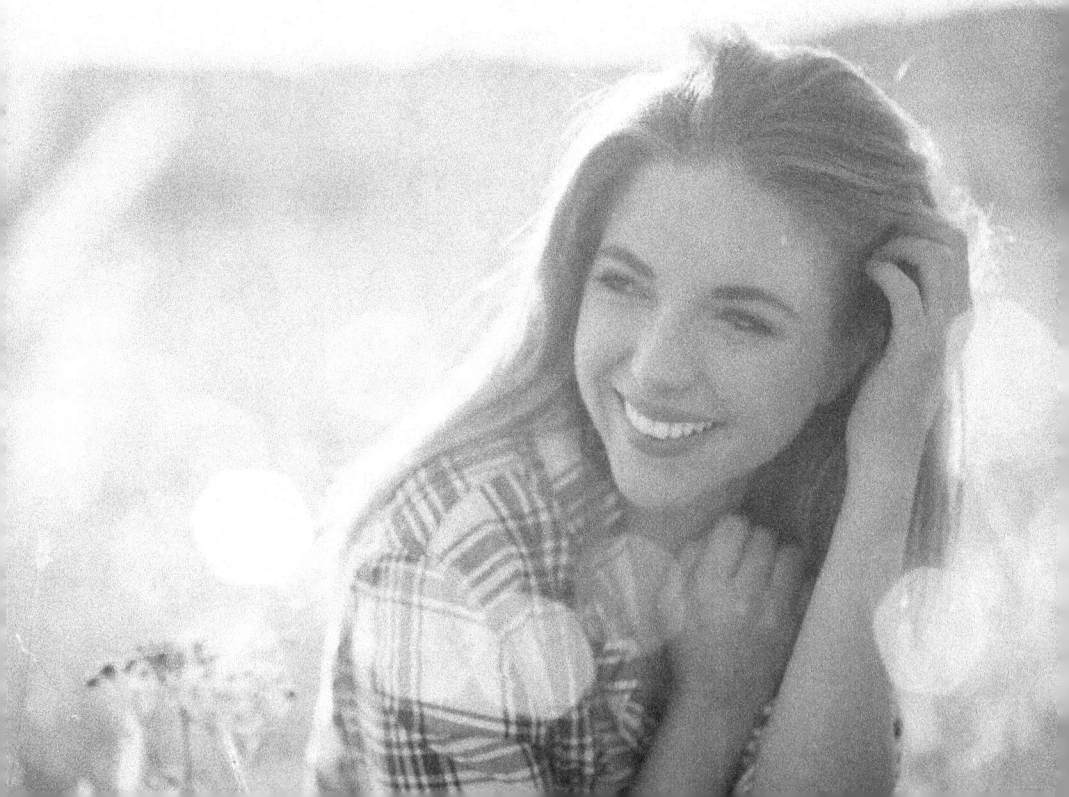

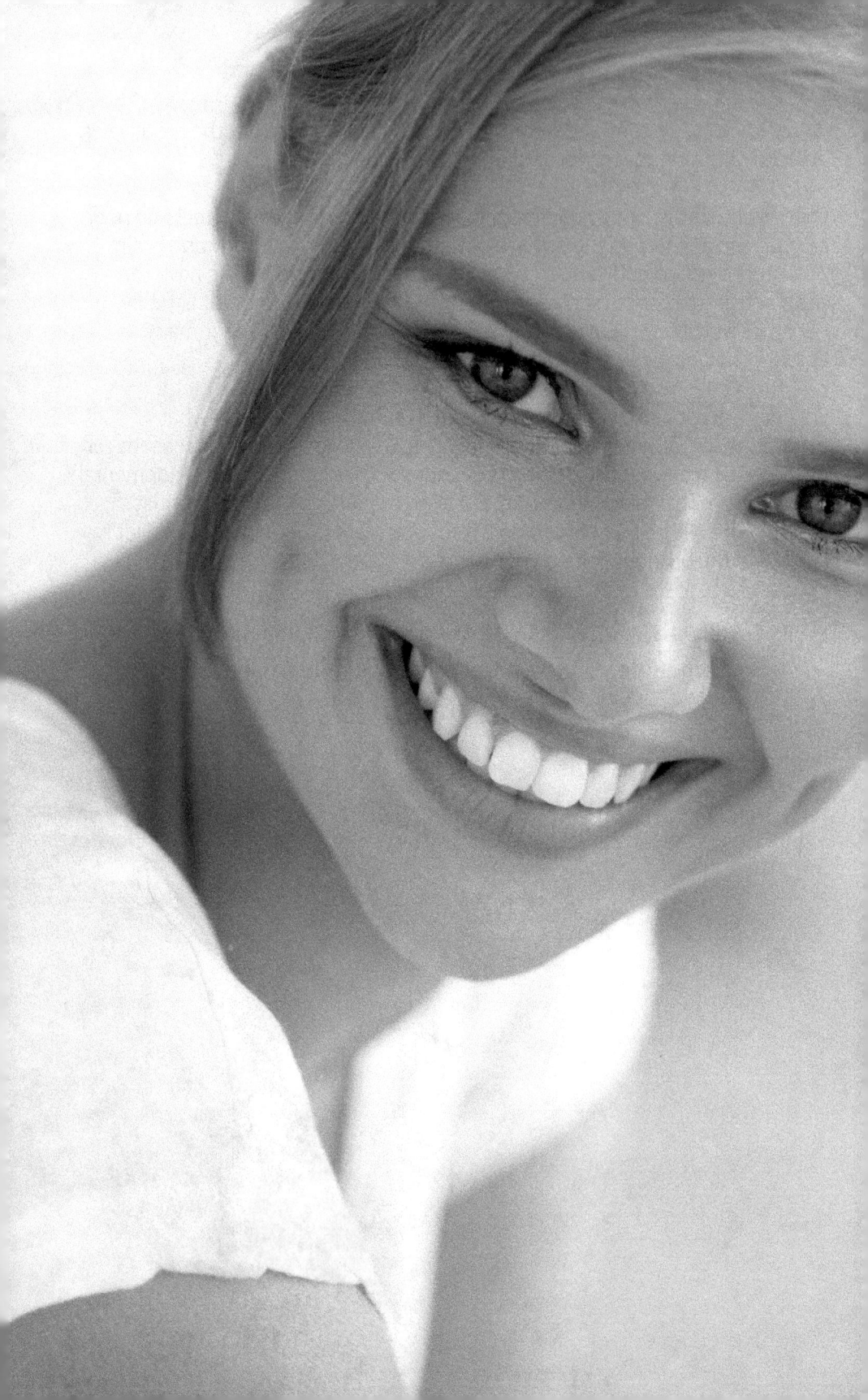

CHAPTER 2

When Should My Child See An Orthodontist?

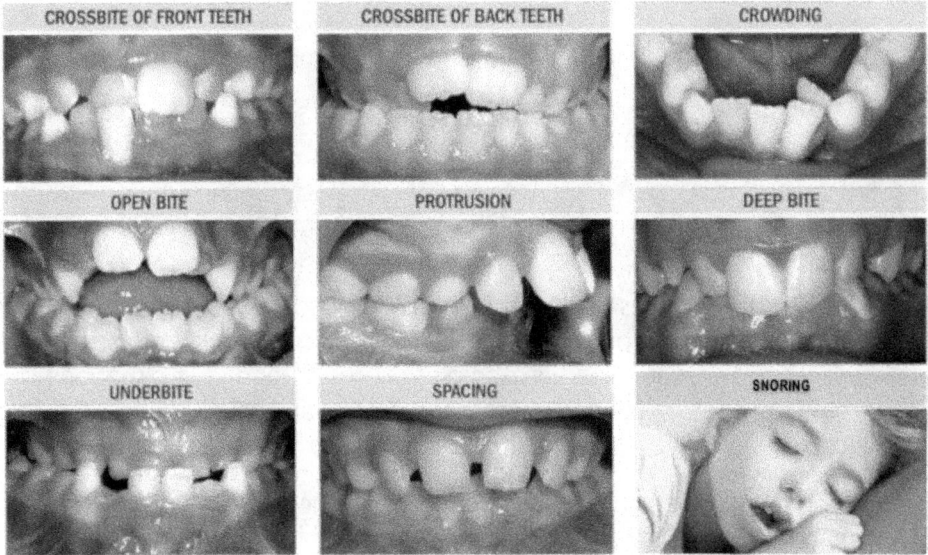

CROSSBITE OF FRONT TEETH

CROSSBITE OF BACK TEETH

CROWDING

OPEN BITE

PROTRUSION

DEEP BITE

UNDERBITE

SPACING

SNORING

Take a look at the pictures above. These are all issues that represent non-ideal bites. Left untreated, they have potential to lead to issues with tooth development, jaw alignment, gum issues, or social concerns. Not all of these problems need orthodontic treatment immediately, but they are worthwhile to at least be *evaluated* by an orthodontist sooner rather than later. What may not look significant to a parent may actually be significant to an orthodontist with experience seeing these types of issues every day.

In order to evaluate what may or may not be concerning, the American Association of Orthodontists recommends that kids have their first orthodontic check-up by a **licensed orthodontist*** starting at age 7 or 8. This recommendation is NOT self-serving. Orthodontists are just looking out for the best interest of your child to avoid serious dental problems and, when indicated, keep treatment easy, painless, and simple.

Going to the orthodontist around your child's 7th birthday is really no different than going to the family dentist for routine dental cleanings or

* All orthodontists are dentists and went to dental school, but your family dentist is not the same as a licensed orthodontist and did not complete the additional training to legally call themselves an orthodontist. They may provide orthodontic services, but they are not an orthodontist. Read on to learn more.

the pediatrician for wellness check-ups. This initial visit is just a checkup to give you peace of mind for what to expect over the next few years! It's just a natural part of child rearing and a smart thing for you to do as a parent, with the orthodontist being the one to evaluate their jaw growth and dental development.

I know what you're thinking right now, and want to make sure something is crystal clear.

> I want you to absolutely realize that seeing the orthodontist at age 7-8 does NOT imply in any way that "braces" will be placed at that visit or treatment will be started/finished sooner.

Please do not think it does! Every child is different so there's no one blanket answer or recommendation with respect to when treatment should begin. However, since all of the previous examples represent non-ideal situations, if you see them or suspect an issue, there's no harm and usually NO COST involved in scheduling a visit with an orthodontist to have them checked out.

In some kids that have significant bite issues, treatment actually IS indicated at a younger age. However, instead of a full set of braces, sometimes a simple appliance to help with jaw positioning or breathing will do the trick. Sometimes just a few braces are placed to move teeth into a better position to avoid gum problems. If treatment is advised, your orthodontist will be able to help you understand timing as well as what tools will be used.

Fortunately, most kids do have good jaw structures, and early intervention isn't needed, or the issues are mild enough to be delayed until later. However, to avoid complications to the other developing teeth, avoid harm to the gums, or avoid poor growth of the jaws it's best to have a professional opinion at age 7 to determine if your child's specific situation warrants attention now or if it can wait.

With that being said, I know many parents see young kids (before middle school age) with braces on their teeth and ask me if braces are, indeed, starting earlier now, since most parents remember having braces on themselves or their friends during the junior high years.

The answer is that "braces", in the sense of fully correcting the bite, cannot be done until all the adult teeth come in the mouth. So, no, the "braces" process to align all the teeth still can't be done until the teenage years. Nothing has changed there.

However, that is the part that deals with only the teeth. What many parents (and some dentists) do not realize is that tooth development alone does not necessarily dictate when the best time is to see an orthodontist. Many kids have issues with either upper or lower jaw development that parents and family dentists CAN'T easily see or may not recognize are even a problem.

If there is an underlying jaw issue, this might be easily addressed when the bones are young, soft, and easily molded. Also, if the bones are set up properly when young, some kids are even lucky enough to not require braces when they are older...and that's pretty cool!

If something actually is indicated for treatment earlier instead of later, corrections done when kids are younger typically are usually easy and painless! This does not mean that braces to fix the teeth aren't going to be needed later, but it does usually mean that the process will be a lot quicker, less expensive, and less invasive!

The goal of seeing kids around age 7 is to make things easy and make sure your child will be in good shape for the years to come! However, even with knowing that they should see an orthodontist between ages 7-8, there are many reasons why parents don't.

1. **Parents do not want to take action, even if they know they should.**
    Out of fear of dentist, concern over costs, distrust of medical professionals from a poor experience in the past, or feeling that seeing an orthodontist when baby teeth are present is "unnecessary", these reasons often are at the core of not scheduling a visit. While many issues may not need addressing now, many problems are subtle and will lead to big problems later. Unfortunately, the optimal time to head off issues with the bite and jaw development has passed once all the adult teeth come in. There should never be a charge for seeing an orthodontist for an initial check-up, so use this as an opportunity to form trust with your provider and ASK QUESTIONS until you are comfortable. It's your child's mouth and orthodontists are here to help. Take advantage of your time with them!

2. **Parents have had poor dental experiences in the past.** There is no room in our profession for those who can't provide you an exceptional patient experience as well as an exceptional smile. While I cannot speak or apologize for the poor experience you may have had, I have not met many providers that truly aren't looking out for your family's best interest first

and foremost. Find an orthodontic specialist that offers not only state of the art technology for your child but state of the art service. Orthodontic specialists should provide every opportunity for patients, especially our younger patients, to feel comfortable, safe, and secure in our care.

3. **Patients are afraid it's going to hurt**. There is nothing that orthodontists will do at an initial visit that will hurt or be uncomfortable for your child. Even if treatment is indicated, modern technology—and choosing the right orthodontist—can ensure that your child enjoys a comfortable and easy orthodontic experience.

4. **Patients are afraid it's going to cost too much.** Not only are most orthodontic procedures more affordable than ever, but dental insurance, flexible payment plans and a variety of other financing options make this all but a moot point for most of my patients. Remember, orthodontists are here to make sure your child's teeth, smile, and jaw are aligned to make his or her life better—period! Most providers are very accommodating with payment plans to ensure a dental issue is not left uncorrected solely due to finances.

5. **Patients are afraid it's going to take too long / miss too much school or work.** Regardless of the type of orthodontic procedure your child needs, time is of the essence. Modern technology and ease of access allows us to work around your child's school schedule with minimal absences. After initial 1-2 visits (which can be up to an hour) most visits after the braces are on last 10-30 minutes...and are typically spaced out 6-12 weeks at a time! There is **NO REASON** any child should have to miss school unless you want them to!

Many parents have the faulty thinking that by doing recommended treatment early their child will have "had braces twice". Thus, they elect to ignore the advice of their orthodontist and erroneously think the orthodontist's goal is just aligning a few crooked teeth or to get money.

They feel that if it's just straightening teeth, then why do it now and "pay twice" if it's going to still need to be done later. *Honestly, I agree 100%.* In my office, I rarely will recommend early (or "Phase I") treatment if strictly for cosmetic issues, unless a child is being bullied or teased because of their smile. (More on that in a subsequent chapter.)

To reiterate: most "early" treatment simply to cosmetically align the front teeth is NOT necessary!

Also some parents put off orthodontic treatment not because they think (or hope) their child will grow out of the problem. I truly wish that was the case, and life would be easier for everyone if it was, but it's unfortunately not.

Issues with your child's bite are not like their tantrums, a bad haircut, or acne. They don't grow out of it. Bite issues do NOT fix themselves and they need intervention to correct. Left alone, these problems often grow worse and harder to resolve.

Therefore, I will often recommend early treatment when there are functional issues and jaw development concerns/jaw size mismatches.

The best way to think of this idea is that there are two parts of the bite that eventually need straightened - the underlying bones (the basement) and the teeth (the house on top). So, straightening the bones early when they are soft sets up the foundation to the right dimensions to accommodate the eventual house which will be built upon it. Then, once all the adult teeth come in later on (during the teenage years), braces to straighten all the teeth will be used.

The reality is that both the bone and tooth aspects will need to be addressed at some point, but breaking it up into two parts is easier on the child and sets up a better environment for the adult teeth to come in.

As a bonus to parents in my office, I often give a comprehensive fee for both the early bone portion and the later tooth portion, so that you'll be fully covered from start to finish. That way there's no feeling any pressure to put on braces on the teeth before the truly appropriate time!

When all the adult teeth come in, some kids have already matured to the point where the window to work with their softer bones has closed. Treatment now becomes much more complicated and could even involve jaw surgery, instead of what may have been a simple fix if the child only had been evaluated earlier.

Even if you're late getting your son or daughter in, it's still possible to provide good treatment options (or even realize they don't even NEED braces!) However, the sooner you know and learn about your options, the better!

Remember that age 7 is the right time to schedule a visit. I hope this was made clear, and that the reasons for doing so are truly in your child's best interest, not "just because"!

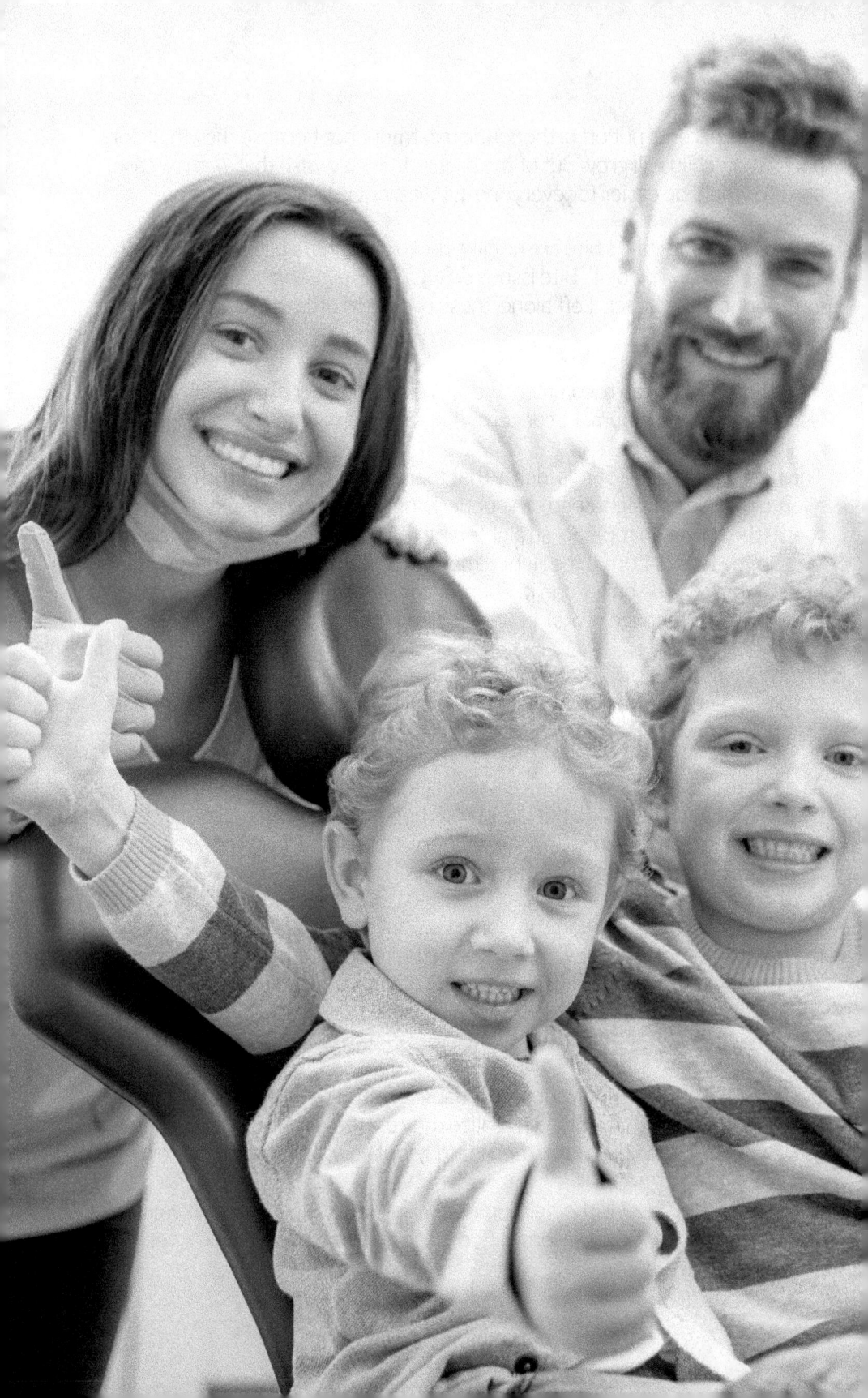

CHAPTER 3

Why an Orthodontist?

You undoubtedly already have a family dentist. But how does an orthodontist differ from your dentist?

Just as the family doctor refers his patients with possible or significant heart disease issues to a cardiologist, and if need be, the cardiologist refers to a surgeon, the best dentists refer patients with orthodontic needs to orthodontists. They don't work alone!

Here are the facts.

All orthodontists actually *are* licensed dentists. Just like your family dentist, we completed 4 years of dental school and are well-versed in basic dental procedures. However, in order to be called an orthodontic specialist, or "orthodontist", the difference is that we also had to complete an additional 2-3 years of a full-time residency where we focused on nothing else other than moving teeth and providing the best treatment for conditions like:

- difficulties chewing or biting
- biting into the cheek, gums, or roof of the mouth
- teeth that meet abnormally or don't meet at all
- teeth grinding or clenching
- crowded, misplaced or blocked out teeth
- early or late loss of teeth
- teeth that protrude
- embarrassing personal appearance due to teeth
- facial imbalances
- teeth or jaw misalignment
- TMJ problems
- chronic headaches and migraines
- poor sleep
- speech difficulties (that may never be outgrown or may develop later)

These are not dental care issues. They are orthodontic issues.

I often get the question from parents who ask "isn't my family dentist also an orthodontist since he sometimes puts braces on people or delivers clear aligners (such as Invisalign®?)" In nearly all instances that is not true. This misconception arises because any dentist can advertise they provide orthodontic services to move teeth, and can do so without qualification or requirement to disclose the amount of training they have (crazy, huh?).

Orthodontists are dental specialists whose ONLY focus is on moving teeth and aligning the jaws to improve our patient's smiles and bites. This is all we do...all day, every day! Yes, we are the guys and gals that use braces and give people "metal mouth" (but we have clear braces too!). Yes we use clear aligners when indicated. Yes, we treat kids and adults. Yes, we give people rubber bands that end up all around the house. Yes, we get made fun of for sometimes using headgear. That's ok, we can handle the jokes because we love the results and smiles we create!

In reality, only 6% of licensed dentists are actually orthodontists who have completed a full-time accredited residency program. Also, nearly everyone who has completed this additional training limits the scope of their practice to just moving teeth, so they can focus their expertise here and get really, really good at doing so. **The bottom line is that all orthodontists are dentists, but not all dentists are orthodontists!**

You may ask, "How do I know my doctor is an orthodontist?" It's a good question and a critical one to ask as you seek additional treatment for your child's dental issues.

One easy way to be sure you are seeing an orthodontic specialist is to look for the seal of membership in the American Association of Orthodontists, as only licensed orthodontic specialists are eligible to join this organization! Visit www.braces.org to ensure your orthodontic provider is a member!

Alternatively, you can ask your doctor if he or she has completed a two- to three-year accredited residency in orthodontics and check with your state dental board to follow up on his reply.

Also, look for the words "dental specialist in orthodontics" or ask your general dentist for a referral to a specialist. In urban and suburban areas, it will take minimal effort to find a specialist. In more remote, rural locations, your search might take you to another city or town. Don't be afraid to ask your dentist if an orthodontist travels to your town every month to see patients. There's a chance an orthodontist from a larger city comes to your town and works out of another dental office once or twice per month. Knowing this information can save valuable driving time.

As you research your options, you may happen to come across one of many non-accredited orthodontic training programs with official-sounding names and important-sounding certifications available to your family dentist. However, they are NOT officially accredited or recognized orthodontic residency programs. Their "graduates" are NOT licensed orthodontists, and these providers cannot legally say they are an orthodontist on their website or in person, although they may say they provide orthodontic services.

There is a subtle, but BIG difference in those terms. Be sure to look up your potential provider's credentials at braces.org, the official website of the AAO, if you are unsure, as only a bonafide, licensed orthodontist will be listed on their site*.

As orthodontists, our #1 objective is to partner with our patients, families, and their family dentist to safely give you an awesome smile...while having a little fun with us on your journey as well. With today's technology, easy financing, and convenient appointment times getting orthodontic treatment by a licensed orthodontist is easier than ever. I've never had ANYONE regret this decision, and doubt that you will either!

> **!** VERY IMPORTANT: Unlike medicine, where you often need a referral from your primary doctor to see a specialist, that is not the case with dentistry! There is NO NEED for a referral from your family dentist in order to schedule an appointment with an orthodontist. You can do this completely on your own.

Great news!

*With that being said, I want you to realize there is no disrespect implied or intended to any dental colleague with the any of the above paragraphs. The words are simply statements of fact. I personally know some family dentists (who are not licensed orthodontists) that actually do very good orthodontic work. Also, I also know licensed orthodontists whose outcomes are consistently questionable (unfortunately every profession has a hierarchy of skills, and it would be unfair for me to say that every orthodontist is top notch).

> **Call us at 484.730.1921 or go to www.coesmiles.com to schedule your own Customized Smile Analysis.**

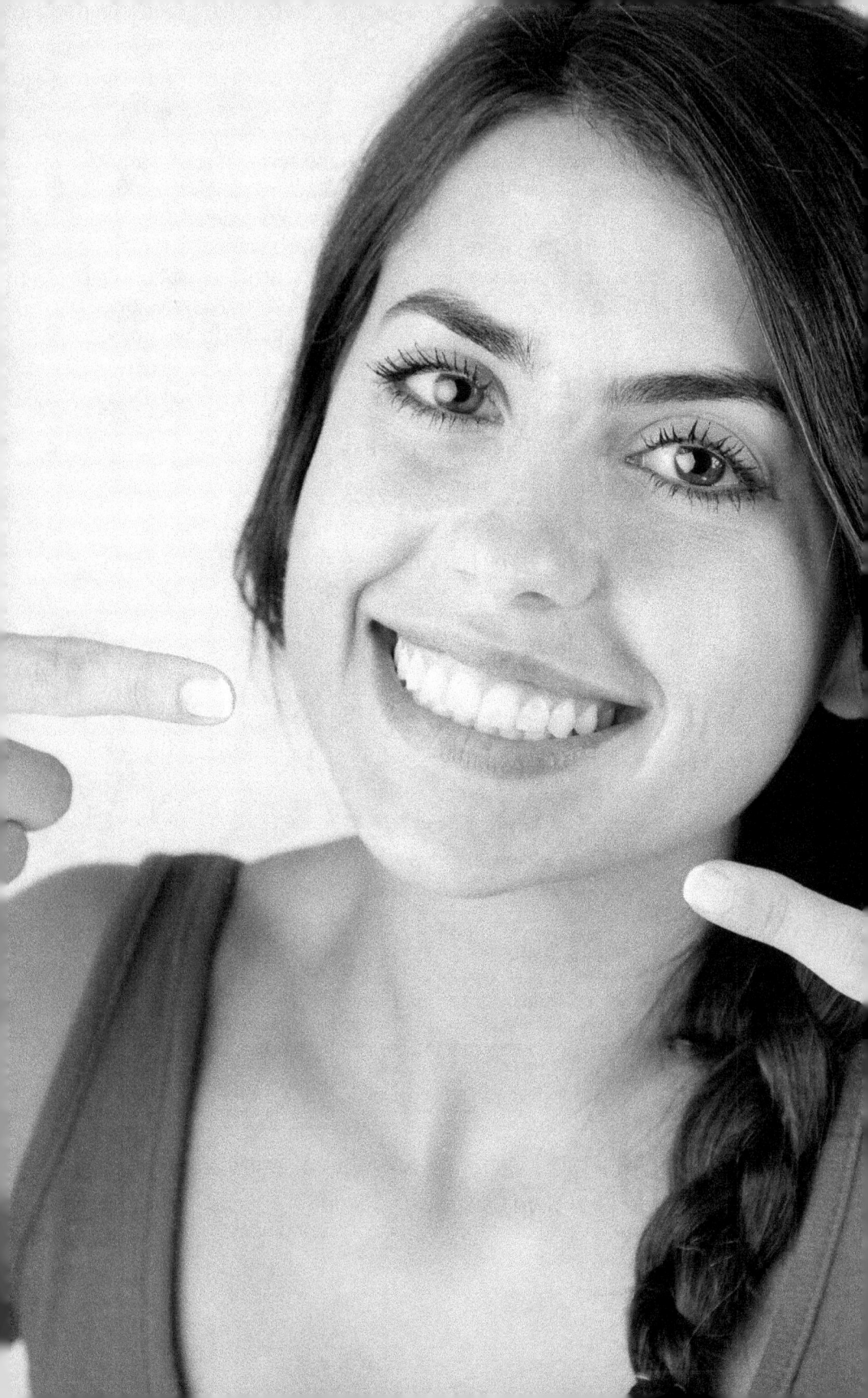

CHAPTER 4

Sleep, Breathing, Orthodontics, and Your Growing Child

Whether we've just been thoroughly exhausted, had a cold, or just slept in a funny position, likely everyone has had a chance to saw a few logs! While most of the time snoring is thought of as an "adult" nighttime activity, sporadic snoring in kids also can occur. Usually this is not anything to be concerned about. However, frequent snoring outside of periods of known sickness or during allergy season could be cause for alarm.

Chronic snoring and chronic mouth-breathing in kids is not "normal", and may indicate a small airway and a higher potential for sleep apnea as an adult. Additionally, research is clear that kids with breathing issues and not getting enough oxygen during sleep hours are prone to a host of negative associations with their body and brain development, including, but not limited to, ADHD, chronic headaches, chronic bed-wetting, and poor performance in school. Other conditions often associated with poor breathing are listed in the chart below. This list does not mean that having one or more of these conditions is absolutely indicative of an underlying breathing issue, but it shouldn't be dismissed either. It's just something to consider as you are speaking with your child's pediatrician and something to ask, as they may not be aware of the link.

As parents, you can do a couple really quick things to help assess if your child may have a suspected breathing issue during sleep. First, ask yourself the following six questions. If you answer "yes" to any of the following, it wouldn't be a bad idea to investigate further.

1. Does my child snore frequently?
2. Does my child usually sleep through the night, awake sleepy, or tire easily?
3. Does my child sound "nasally" when speaking?
4. Does my child have problems focusing in school?
5. Does my child grind his/her teeth?
6. Does my child get frequent headaches?

Secondly, take a look in your child's mouth and have them say "AHHHHH".

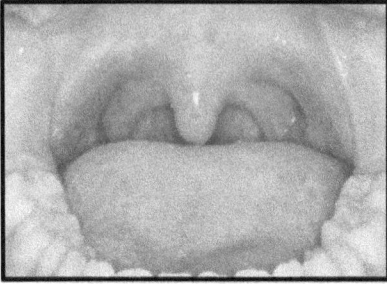

Normal Tonsils

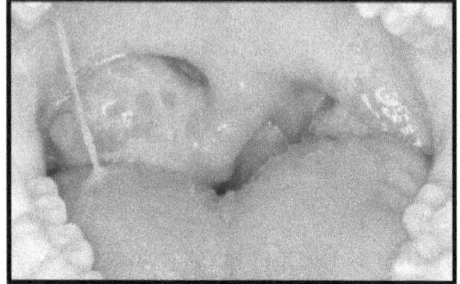

Severely Enlarged Tonsils

Look at the size of their tonsils. It should look like the picture on the left, which is normal. If you notice something that looks more like the right picture, this is NOT NORMAL and your child could be at serious risk for breathing issues.

The following images represent "normal" airways. For the normal patients, you can see how wide open the airway is from the nose all the way down.

Normal Airways

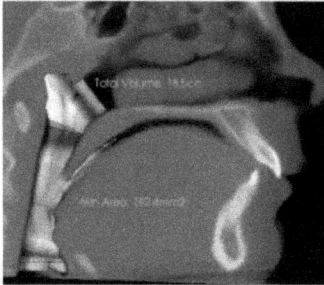

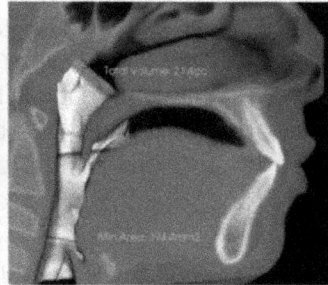

Concerning Airways

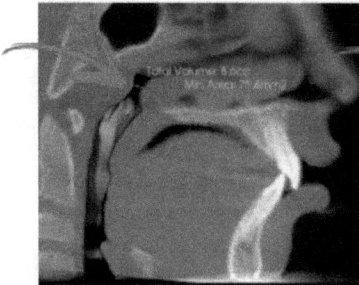

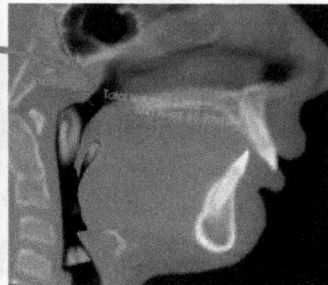

In contrast, these two images represent "concerning" airways. You should easily be able to see the difference in these examples vs. those above. Of note is the swelling of the adenoids (at the tip of the arrow) constricting the airway and making it hard to breathe. Both of the patients below reported poor breathing through their nose and frequent snoring at night.

So, you may be now asking, what does this have to do with orthodontics? What are braces going to do about it?

Actually, braces themselves will do very little. It's not about braces at all. As part of an orthodontic check-up when kids are 7-8, looking at the airway and asking parents questions about their child's sleep habits are a critical piece of the puzzle. A child's smile, jaw development, and tooth eruption often follows, and is affected by, the way the child breathes.

Orthodontists, if they see children early enough (such as age 7-8, or earlier, as previously recommended!) can appropriately evaluate and suggest an approach, if indicated, to help get children breathing better and minimize any detrimental impacts on their growth and life.

I often find that a child's pediatrician does recognize breathing issues, but may not be as sensitive to the nature of kids' airways on the overall growth of their jaws as an orthodontist is. Orthodontists are able to change the structures of the jaws, including those that surround your child's airway. This aspect is what orthodontists CAN measure and evaluate, and are the specialists for doing so!

Many breathing issues are associated with small upper jaws. Therefore, making the jaw size "normal" through orthodontic means when kids are young has tons of benefits.

1. It's easy and painless. Kids' bones are really soft when young, so there's not a lot of discomfort to do so.

2. Many issues related to sleep and poor breathing may improve just by normalizing the jaw size.

3. If this conservative solution with orthodontics solves this issue, then you eliminate the need for medications or surgical procedures (that still don't address the underlying structural problem).
4. If the jaws are small to begin with, at the very worst they will now be the right size and allow for the adult teeth to come in better and with more room, regardless of effect on breathing. At the very best, there will be room for the teeth AND the breathing issues will also be eliminated.

These are all "wins" for the child (as well as mom and dad) in my book!

Now, I would be irresponsible to say that improving jaw size with kids is going to solve or be part of the solution for every breathing issue. It absolutely will not. Regardless, correcting the jaw structures early will show what effect the small jaws have (or do not have) on breathing, and will ultimately help the child's medical team better focus their efforts on what issues may remain.

Orthodontists have many tools to help conservatively evaluate and treat kids with suspected issues, and will work closely with the child's pediatrician to provide a comprehensive solution. Unfortunately, by waiting for your child to "outgrow" the problem or waiting to see the orthodontist until all the adult teeth have come in, as is commonly suggested, is often too late to conservatively reverse any developmental issues that may have arose due to poor breathing.

This chapter is not meant to scare you as parents, as many kids truly do not have any breathing issues, especially not those related to orthodontics. However, since an orthodontist can easily let you know if there is an issue with a quick check-up, and there usually not a charge to do so, it doesn't hurt to be proactive and get your child evaluated (especially if YOU are noticing an issue)!

Call us at 484.730.1921 or go to www.coesmiles.com to schedule your own Customized Smile Analysis.

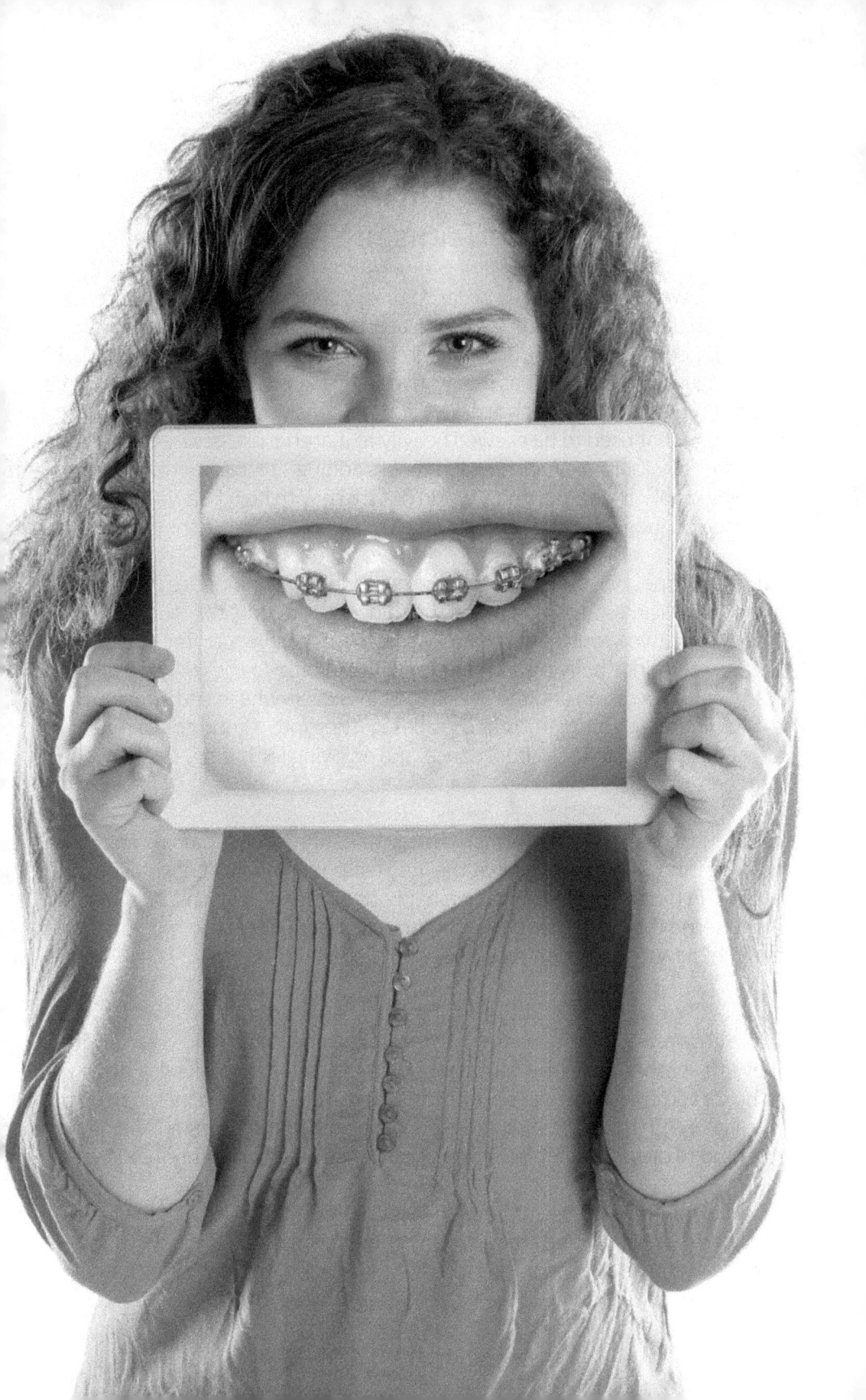

CHAPTER 5

Smiles, Social Media, and Life Beyond The Teenage Years

When we were growing up, in order to think you were "cool", you wanted to hang with the "popular" kids, wear the latest fashions (Skidz, Chuck Taylors, and crimped hair anyone?), or be the first to have the latest He-Man or Barbie action figures. Not much has really changed except the clothing brand names and the types of toys...which are now more expensive and more electronic! However, what used to be skewed heavily to material pressures, there's now Facebook, Instagram, Snapchat, and others adding severe emotional pressure to being "cool". It's a whole new world out there with how kids validate themselves, judge their self-worth, and try to find out where they "fit in".

Whether or not we agree with it as parents, we and our kids are now in an age of selfies and social media, and the things my patients tell me that go on in school today were once unthinkable in my mind growing up. Teen suicide has skyrocketed since bullying and social media shaming rose to ugly prominence. Also, teen depression and the desire to fit in is everywhere and affects everything from getting the good grades, getting into a good college, getting a first date, going to the school dance, and enjoying (or hating) their childhood and teen years.

I feel, due to the ease of information dissemination, social shaming and bullying is now a lot worse, or, at the very least, more prevalent. Maybe not "worse" in the sense of how often it happens or for the reasons, but "worse" in the sense that more people know about it, more people can "pile-on" easier, and the "news" spreads so much faster.

You used to have to wait until lunchtime or even days later to hear about the latest gossip, but now it becomes instant with a few clicks, and you can't just move to another table or leave the room. Spats and personal tussles that used to be forgotten in a few days now persist and are archived indefinitely on the internet. With the hours that kids spend on social media apps and on devices, it is hard to distance one's self from the barrage and constant reminders.

Also, bullying used to be confined to face-to-face interaction and limited to just a few people. However, behind a computer screen and in off-school hours, even normally reserved kids can turn into keyboard warriors and it can get far nastier than most would dare in person. Most importantly and dangerously, the interactions can be viewed by many people simultaneously and this sudden volume of negative attention can be overwhelming.

Often, the teenage mind has not developed enough to handle these pressures and cope effectively like an adult would. Teens can internalize this desire to fit in, and a sense of embarrassment or helplessness can quickly spiral out of control.

Unfortunately, many cases of teen suicide share one thing in common: shocked and bewildered parents who could not conceive of their child ending his own life due to seemingly "insignificant" things going on in social situations that they were never even aware of happening. Sure, parents might notice their child was a little depressed. They knew he was being bullied and spending more time home, alone and not leaving his room, but he is a teenager and this just a part of growing up and developing your tougher skin, right?

The below list is not all inclusive, but are just some things to become aware of as a parent. Regardless of how you may think these things are "just a phase" or "shall pass" the best thing to do is talk with your child. You'd be surprised about what they may tell you if they just ask!

Signs Your Child May Be Being Bullied

- decrease in self-esteem
- not wanting to go to school
- skipping school
- injuries they can't explain
- self-destructive behaviors (e.g., harming themselves)
- declining school grades
- sleep difficulties
- loss of interest in schoolwork or activities
- sudden loss of friends or avoiding social groups
- changes in eating habits

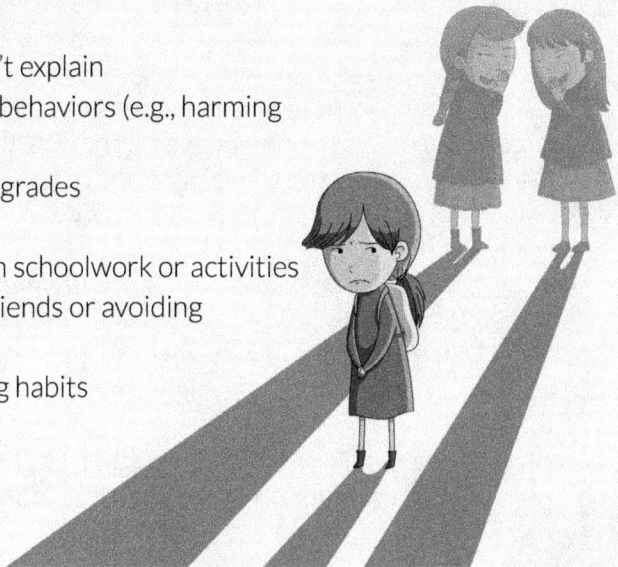

"Ok," you may be asking, "so what does all of this have to do with orthodontics?" Well, actually a lot.

Sometimes, kids bully or tease each other for no reason, and having teeth that stick out, having a huge underbite, or just being a little different looking is enough to incite and escalate the situation.

Great smiles go incredibly far in improving one's self-image and projecting self-confidence. While a great smile itself will not prevent bullying from occurring (there's no one that can say that), just having a child that is prouder of themselves and realizes their higher self-worth at baseline can help provide a good foundation to cope with these pressures should they come.

Bullies are cowards and tend to prey on who they perceive as weak and insecure in order to make themselves feel better. Those kids who project security, self-worth, and confidence with a great smile on their face* are less likely to fall victim or be a target, and that's a real win in my book!

Beyond high school and surviving the teenage years, though, there's a life ahead of your child. Going on college admission interviews, dating and finding a partner, seeking employment, trying to fit into new workplaces all require confidence, security, and self-esteem! Additionally, the goals of most parents include providing as good of a life as possible for their kids.

Think about what happens with the college decision process. Parents know that it's not about the few years of college and what happens in the classroom, but rather the network and experiences their kids will have during those years that will help shape the forty or fifty years afterward. Therefore, parents just about kill themselves over their kids' college admissions, starting the process younger and younger, encouraging activities that will "look good" to programs, trekking around the country on campus visits, enrolling their kids in college admission test prep classes, and taking on serious debt in hopes the investment in their education will pay off for with a good/better future for their kids!

Your child's smile is no different.

However, unlike the uncertainty with what will happen after college, there are certain and known benefits that a straight smile has on improved health!

No parent wants their child to suffer, and bite issues have been linked to chronic headaches, migraines, digestive problems, poor sleep in adults.

Often, when kids have these issues the mouth is the last place we as parents check – and sometimes it is even overlooked by physicians as a contributor as well!

Visiting an orthodontist now can help recognize issues that might be easily corrected and help avoid significant problems later in life. Orthodontic treatment isn't just fixing a cosmetic issue. This is an investment in your child's future health.

*Please do not misinterpret the purpose of this chapter. We all know that crooked teeth and a poor smile are not the only aspects or physical traits where teasing can occur. That would be extremely short-sighted and naïve to assume, as well as over-simplifying an incredibly complex emotional, mental, and physical process. However, if a better smile can give a child increased confidence and increased self-esteem to let their individual personalities shine, express their talents, and stand up to bullies for themselves, then all the better!

Call us at 484.730.1921 or go to www.coesmiles.com to schedule your own Customized Smile Analysis.

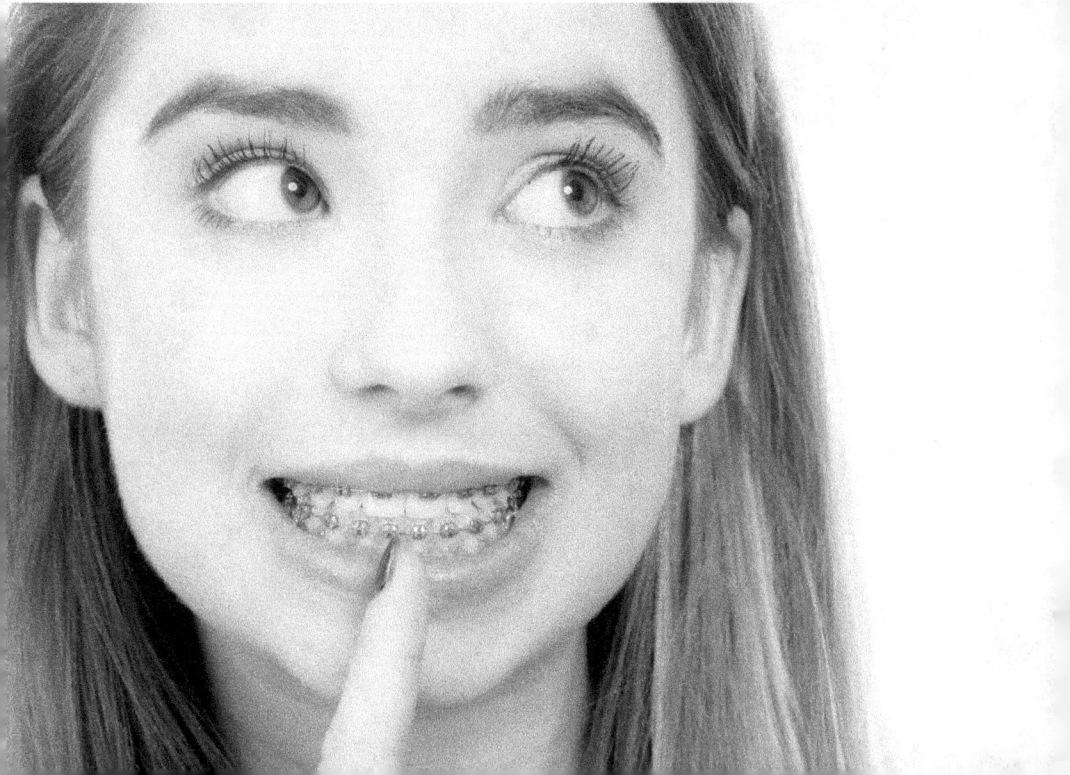

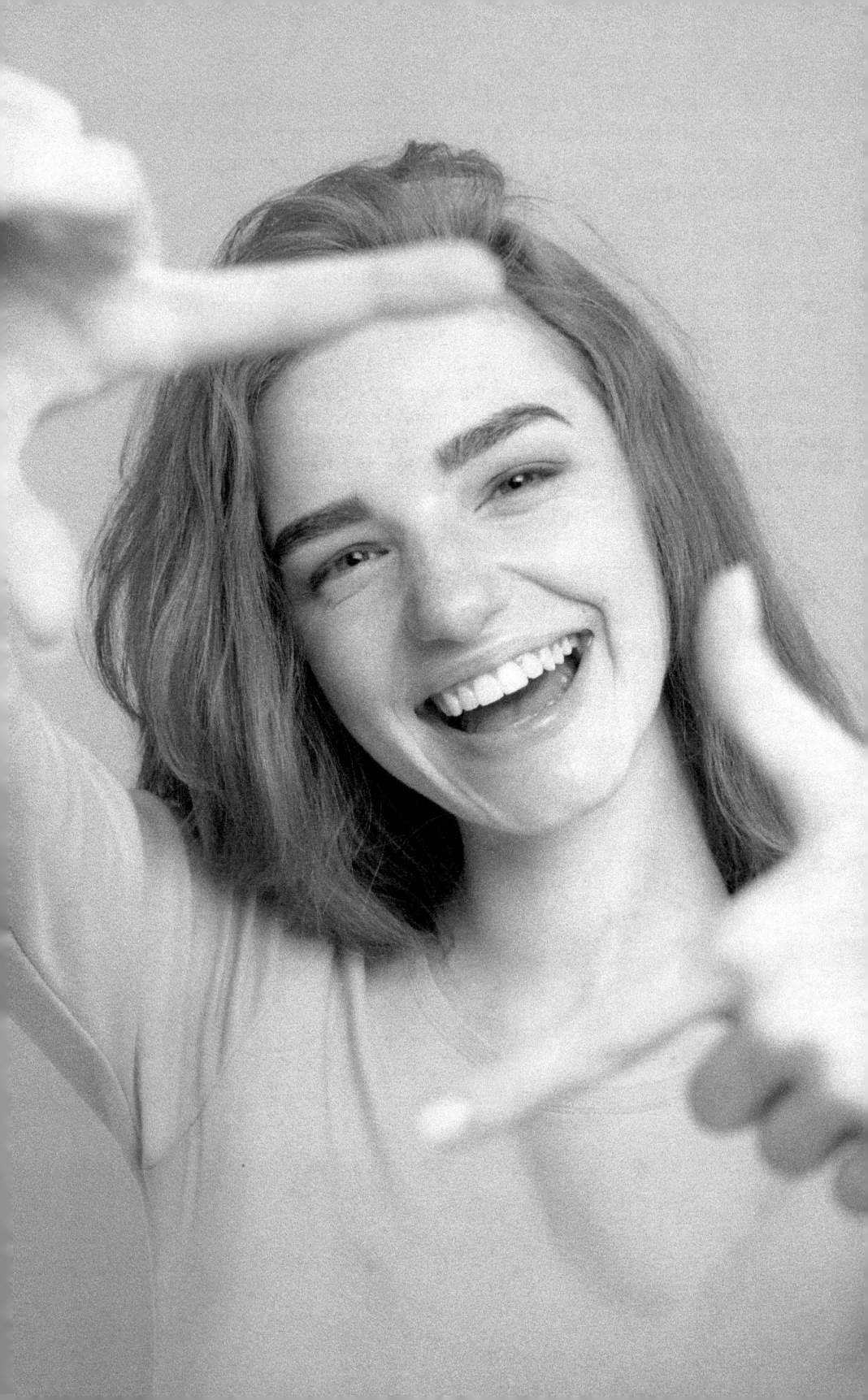

CHAPTER 6

How To Confidently Choose an Orthodontist

Now that you know why you should see an orthodontist, and how orthodontics can help your child, you need to find a doctor! With the number of providers likely available in your area, how do you know who you should trust for your family's smiles? (Hint: Not all orthodontists are the same!)

Orthodontics goes way beyond simply putting on braces or handing out clear aligners. Honestly, with enough practice, anyone can learn how take some glue and stick a brace on a tooth, digitally set up teeth on a computer, or just click a button to approve treatment. Those mechanical acts actually are not difficult!

What is difficult finding someone that can do it correctly, knows what moving a tooth to a certain spot means, knows how that placement affects the overall result you want, effectively communicates that knowledge to you as the parent, and makes the entire experience exceptional. In other words, you need a **trustworthy advisor that can be trusted**.

While there are lots of options for orthodontic treatment out there, this process is an investment both in time and money. You only want to do it once, and you want to be sure you are getting the best team for the job!

Once families hear or realize they should have their child see an orthodontist, often the first place they go to look for information is on the internet, and, honestly, that's where I would go first as well. By searching for "orthodontist in (your town)", you'll likely get choice of several offices as well as links to their Google reviews. These are a great starting point. An orthodontic office's success is built on a backbone of ethics and earned trust. Therefore, you'll want to look for honest, well-written reviews that discuss a patient's specific experience in specific detail, not in generalities. These will give you nice insight into the office, especially if the sentiments are consistent!

A word of caution about online reviews: some unethical providers will have their friends, staff, or others write reviews to just "pad" their numbers, or, worse, use 3rd party sites to "boost" the number of reviews but the reviews will not actually provide any text or helpful information. These methods to game the system can often be picked out easily and should be discounted.

If the office is questionable with their ethics in getting reviews and confusing with their outward appearance to the public, it likely won't be any better once you are a patient!

Also, some providers may have 1-star reviews. Don't dismiss this or think they are a "bad" office. Go read them, as they are valuable information. An occasional negative review is not a bad thing and just shows they are human. No office can please everyone, and reading those negative reviews can give you a lot of insight. A quick read can easily tell you whether that review is "credible" or if it is a one-off rant by an unreasonable person. If so, and they are isolated, the office may have had a bad day or there was a misunderstanding. However, if there are multiple poor reviews consistently highlighting the same concerns, you may want to avoid that office.

Once you read reviews, you'll likely check out a few websites to see the differences among the providers. Here you will want to look for which office best provides answers to your questions and has a warm, friendly feel. If the office took the effort to be helpful and let their personality show on their website (instead of just using stock content), this is usually a good indication your experience with that office will also be good!

After you narrow your choice to the provider you feel would best fit your family's needs and ideals, the next step is to schedule an appointment with that office and meet the team! This the time to then get all your questions ready for them to answer.

The following 10 questions are really common ones parents ask me about my own office, and ones I feel are worthwhile to get solid answers for no matter where you go:

1. Are you a licensed orthodontic specialist?
2. How many cases like mine have you treated before?
3. How do you determine what treatment is beneficial for my case?
4. Are you actively involved with any teaching, lecturing, or current research projects?
5. Do you offer customized, flexible financing options and payment plans with no-interest?
6. Is the initial visit complimentary?
7. How often will I have to miss school or work during the process?
8. What will my experience be like with your team?
9. Do you offer options besides just metal braces for treatment?
10. Would you do the same recommended treatment on your own family member if they had the same issues?

By having these questions answered to your satisfaction, this will be a quick test that you likely are getting a well-qualified team to give your child the best smile in the safest, most efficient, most convenient, and most FUN way possible...because, really, that's what this journey is all about!

Let's go into each of these into more detail.

1. Are you a licensed orthodontic specialist?

The answer should be YES - hands-down, absolutely, no questions asked, no hesitation, and with no other qualification – just YES! Plain and simple.

Moving teeth and working with jaw structures are the only things licensed orthodontists do. We don't perform cleanings. We don't fill cavities. We don't remove wisdom teeth. We don't make dentures. We ONLY correct mis-alignment of the teeth and jaws on kids and adults.

As mentioned in a previous chapter, an easy way to figure out if a provider is an orthodontic specialist is to look for the seal of the American Association of Orthodontists (AAO). Only licensed orthodontic specialists can belong to the AAO and only those who have completed an accredited residency program beyond dental school training can legally call themselves orthodontists.

It's often hard to tell the difference in the potential for a good result or a good provider based on qualifications alone, since no two cases or situations are exactly alike.

Getting a "YES!" to this first question is a good start, but the additional questions below will help differentiate your provider choices and give you clarity with making your decision on who you should trust for your family's orthodontic needs.

2. How many cases like mine have you treated before?

A well-experienced team should be able to provide examples and results of similar cases to your child's that they personally have treated to help put you at ease. Also, a well-qualified doctor will have a nice library of their own results on hand to show you how their treatment of a roughly similar bite to your child's turned out. Once a provider has been in practice for a number of years, common bite issues tend to show up over and over, and the doctor should have these results available to show you and back up their proposed plans.

Fortunately, truly bizarre and unique orthodontic issues are rare. You will be hard pressed to have an experienced doctor say that he or she "hasn't quite seen something like this before". Therefore, it's a good sign you are in good hands if your provider can quickly show you how similar bites to your child's finished well. At the very least, these examples will help you realize that your child's treatment and situation isn't their first rodeo.

If you are shown "stock" examples or, worse, case examples treated by someone else, do not hesitate to ask to see the doctor's own case results or ask if they have the experience to treat an issue like your child's. You have every right to know this. If the doctor does not have examples of your child's exact situation readily available, it does NOT mean they are unqualified. If that is the case, you should just ask if you can see results of other cases they have treated to get a sense of how their smiles look after the braces are removed.

3. How do you determine what treatment is beneficial for my case?

The orthodontist and their team should provide a thorough, individualized analysis of the proposed plan using images (x-rays) and/or models, not just looking in the mouth. You deserve the extra attention this process affords to make your child's smile journey totally customized!

Two of the biggest treatment concerns from parents, and most of the second opinion consultations I do, involve wondering if removal of adult teeth is necessary or if jaw procedures need to happen to get a nice smile for their child. For most cases, removal of adult teeth or jaw surgery is not needed (so you can take a deep sigh of relief now!), but often times when they are, the reasons for doing so were not communicated clearly to the family by the previous orthodontist, thus triggering the second opinion.

My wish in an ideal world would be to never have to recommend these procedures to parents either, but, unfortunately, the world is not ideal and we are all unique human beings. Depending on the smile goals for your child, sometimes things beyond just braces are indicated to keep your child's smile healthy for their lifetime. Doing otherwise may be dangerous, irresponsible, or just not look good. There's no "one size fits all" solution for every patient, and your family is no different! Therefore, if extractions and/or jaw procedures are indicated to reach your goals, you should clearly understand WHY they would be beneficial and have options as well as pros/cons of doing/not doing so reviewed with you.

Since these are the two most common orthodontic "fears" of parents, some office marketing pitches and websites try to play into these concerns to generate business. They do this under the guise of false hope to get your attention and get you in their door, so be cautious of any suggestions with this intent.

During your research, you may also come across websites with slick marketing pitches that suggest using a certain brand of braces or appliances will help avoid removing teeth or even sometimes avoid jaw surgery (or orthodontics!) in the future.   You may even seek out one of the "exclusive" providers on their website for this reason.

Beware of any office that says they never recommend removing adult teeth, never recommend procedures on the jaws, or say they never/only use a certain appliance to avoid having to recommend either of the above. If they've treated more than one orthodontic case in their lifetime, the provider would realize that these statements are absolutely impossible unless every case that would benefit from these procedures is simply referred out of their office and they don't have to treat them!

Also, beware of any office that suggests their treatment is "superior" because they use a specific tool, appliance, or exclusive/revolutionary methods that "traditional" orthodontists do not use or recognize (especially if it is suggested to prevent problems that your child does not or is not at risk to actually have!)

Yes, unfortunately, this stuff goes on in some offices, and less honest practitioners will often play heavily on parent's fears and emotions just to get the "sale".

> ! Fact: all orthodontists have the same access to all the tools/methods, and every orthodontist could use them as they see fit.

If these "revolutionary" techniques were truly that good, everyone would use them, but clearly every orthodontist does not! If this type of "sales pitch" is ever proposed to you, or your parenting sense feels that a certain treatment method sounds too good to be true, it probably is.

> **Remember this:** an appliance or technique is just a tool in the orthodontist's toolbox to get your child a great smile. You would not care to ask your hair stylist which brand of scissors they use, your plumber which brand of pipe sealant they use, or your surgeon which brand of hip replacement they use. You just want the result, safely and efficiently, regardless of what is used to get there. Orthodontics is no different! The braces and appliances should be the brand choices the orthodontist feels comfortable using and this choice should be left to your provider. These tools inherently do not have a brain and are not treating your child, the orthodontist using them is. Let the orthodontist feel comfortable using the tools they are comfortable using!

Having been in practice for many years and been there/seen it/used that, **I can promise you with a 100% straight face and looking you directly in the eyes, that NO appliance or technique is a substitute for an appropriate diagnosis and an individualized, conservative treatment plan.**

Do not hesitate to exercise your right as a parent and ask as many questions as possible (or seek a second opinion) until you feel comfortable that a proposed plan is truly beneficial and, most importantly, appropriate for your child!

Again, please remember...there is no one-size-fits-all solution for everyone (nor can a certain brace brand or appliance manipulate Mother Nature better than another). Your child is unique and should be treated as such.

Whatever plan is proposed, it should meet 100% of your needs in the most conservative way possible, and you should be 100% comfortable that the reasons for doing so were explained clearly by your orthodontist. I cannot stress this sentiment enough! If you are not comfortable or are confused, do NOT start treatment with that office...and seek a second opinion!

4. Are you actively involved with any teaching, lecturing, or current research projects?

Orthodontists that stay up-to-date with continuing education, or better yet, are the ones that provide the education through authoring books, writing scientific articles, or lecture to other doctors are usually abreast of the latest innovations and techniques in orthodontics.

Doctors that lecture are held accountable for their material by their peers, so they often will look deep at their own work and methods to ensure their presentations are truthful and accurate - which then translates to improved care for your family!

Additionally, orthodontic offices that participate with research projects, either independently or in conjunction with a university, show that they are constantly learning and seeking out better ways to deliver care for their patients. This mindset is wonderful to have, and should make you comfortable to know your doctor is constantly looking for better ways to great smiles! If you get asked to participate in a project by your doctor, this should be considered a great honor and you should be very comfortable knowing they are seeking to improve the entire orthodontic profession!

5. Do you offer customized, flexible financing options and payment plans?

The answer should be YES! There should not be any reason why getting a great smile should not be made affordable for every family's budget. Rigid payment terms, credit checks, and budget-stretching monthly payments need to be things of the past. Today's families need and demand financial flexibility, so your orthodontist should give you options to customize the payment structure to best fit your needs. There will be more on this in an upcoming chapter.

6. Is the initial visit complimentary?

It should be!

I realize that some orthodontists still do charge a nominal fee in order to reserve the time for an initial visit with them. That is their choice to do so, and I respect it. However, I've realized that a small charge just to meet with them will never make or break an office's balance sheet and, to me, starts the relationship off with a money-focused mindset instead of being patient and results-focused. Some practitioners may disagree with me, but I see these nickel-and-diming "fees" as just a barrier to potentially helping as many people as possible, and promote exclusion rather than inclusion.

I honestly believe you should have total freedom to evaluate the doctor and the team without any mental pressure or financial strings attached to do so, and extending this courtesy (with imaging included) at the beginning should speak volumes and set the tone for how the rest of the journey will go!

7. How often will I have to miss school or work during the process?

Office hours should be convenient for your schedule to minimize any out of school time or time away from work.

From what I've observed in multiple offices, nothing is more frustrating and creates more friction between the staff and parents than struggling to schedule orthodontic visits around work schedules while trying to also juggle school and other activities your kids are involved in!

Today's orthodontic treatments often allow for extended intervals up to 8-12 weeks between visits, unlike in the past where patients were typically seen every 4 weeks. The actual appointment interval is up to the provider and will vary depending on what is being done, but in general, the appointment intervals are increasing!

An office that is truly patient-centered will likely have evening/weekend hours and not place restrictions on how/when you can be seen for visits. Since every office is different, though, be sure to ask about their policy for appointments to make sure the visits are able to fit your lifestyle before you get started!

8. What will my experience be like with your team?

There is a unique human being attached to those 28 teeth! You should never feel like you are in a "factory" or just a "number" at anyone's office. Every office has a unique experience and does things differently, so it is impossible to suggest or imply what your experience "should" be like, other than it needs to make you feel special. The specifics are a great question to ask your potential doctor!

Also, it is extremely easy to pull up ratings and reviews from patients describing their experience with a certain orthodontist. Simply go to Google and search for orthodontist reviews and ratings in your town and read the testimonials for yourself.

9. Do you offer options besides just metal braces for treatment?

The answer should be absolutely! There are a number of options to move the teeth available now that are esthetic and discreet, but traditional metal braces are still the most common choice for and by kids. Options such as clear aligners, tooth-colored braces that blend in, and braces behind the teeth also are popular and will be discussed in a later chapter.

10. Would you do the same recommended treatment on your own family member if they had the same issues?

If this is not an immediate and un-hesitating YES, then you should definitely seek a second opinion! This is a non-negotiable in my mind without any grey area! Any provider that would recommend a treatment method for YOUR child that they wouldn't do to their OWN family member is not someone I would trust. Period, and I mean, PERIOD.

After reading these 10 questions, you may have ones that weren't answered here (but may be answered elsewhere in the book). However, the actual questions you need to have answered aren't ones I suggest, but are the ones that matter most to you and your child.

So, maybe there should be a bonus #11...

11. Does the doctor have patience with you, is happy to answer any and all questions, and make you feel 100% satisfied that you are making a good decision for your child?

If you ever feel like you were just rushed through their process without ample opportunity to have your questions answered, or felt you were an inconvenience to a doctor's day, you, without any doubt, should seek a second opinion! There is absolutely no reason to ever feel that you and your child aren't the most important person in the orthodontist's world at that moment whenever you visit with them, especially if you don't get that vibe on the initial visit! What do you think is going to happen a year or so down the road?

Additionally, be wary of anyone that belittles other doctors to "pump themselves up" or describes accepted methods other doctors may use for treatment as "old-fashioned" or "outdated". These discussions are childish and have no place in the realm of professionalism or bearing on your child. There are dozens of ways to accomplish a beautiful orthodontic result. NO ONE has the answer for the ONLY right way.

Your conversation with the doctor should only be on what they are going to do to help your child. If the conversation shifts or becomes unprofessional, you have every right to ask them to get it back on track and refocus.

Starting orthodontic treatment is a BIG decision and should never be taken lightly or for granted by any doctor or their team. Your family and their dental well-being is too important for you to ever feel uncomfortable, even for a second.

Make certain you get all your questions answered by the orthodontist or practice's treatment coordinator. Don't hold back. Put them on the spot. Be assertive – it's your family's well being at stake.

In this chapter, I've tried to highlight common concerns from parents and patients, and even some concerns that aren't explicitly asked but I know are going through their minds. My own goal is to have every patient and every patient's parent fully knowledgeable about every aspect of the treatment so that they have zero anxiety. However, if you have a specific concern not answered anywhere in this book, or have a personal and confidential question, you can—with compete assurance of privacy and courtesy—email me directly at drtamburrino@coesmiles.com. I'm happy to respond to you personally if it will help you make a good decision for your family.

> **Call us at 484.730.1921 or go to www.coesmiles.com
> to schedule your own Customized Smile Analysis.**

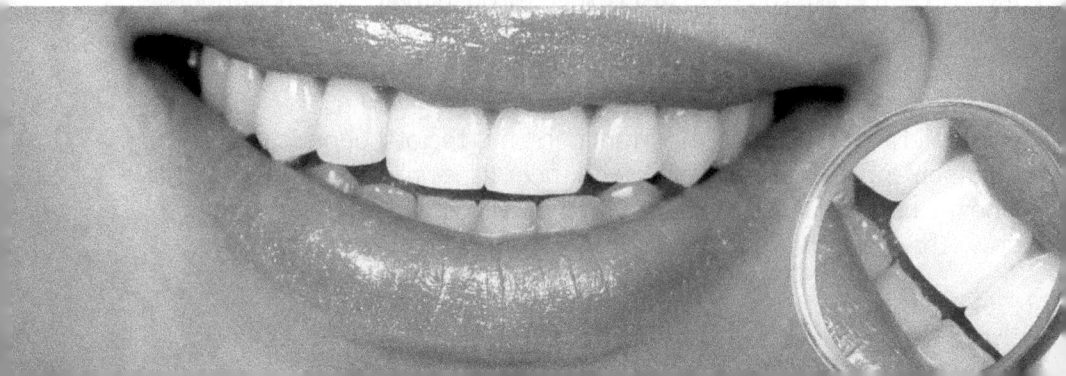

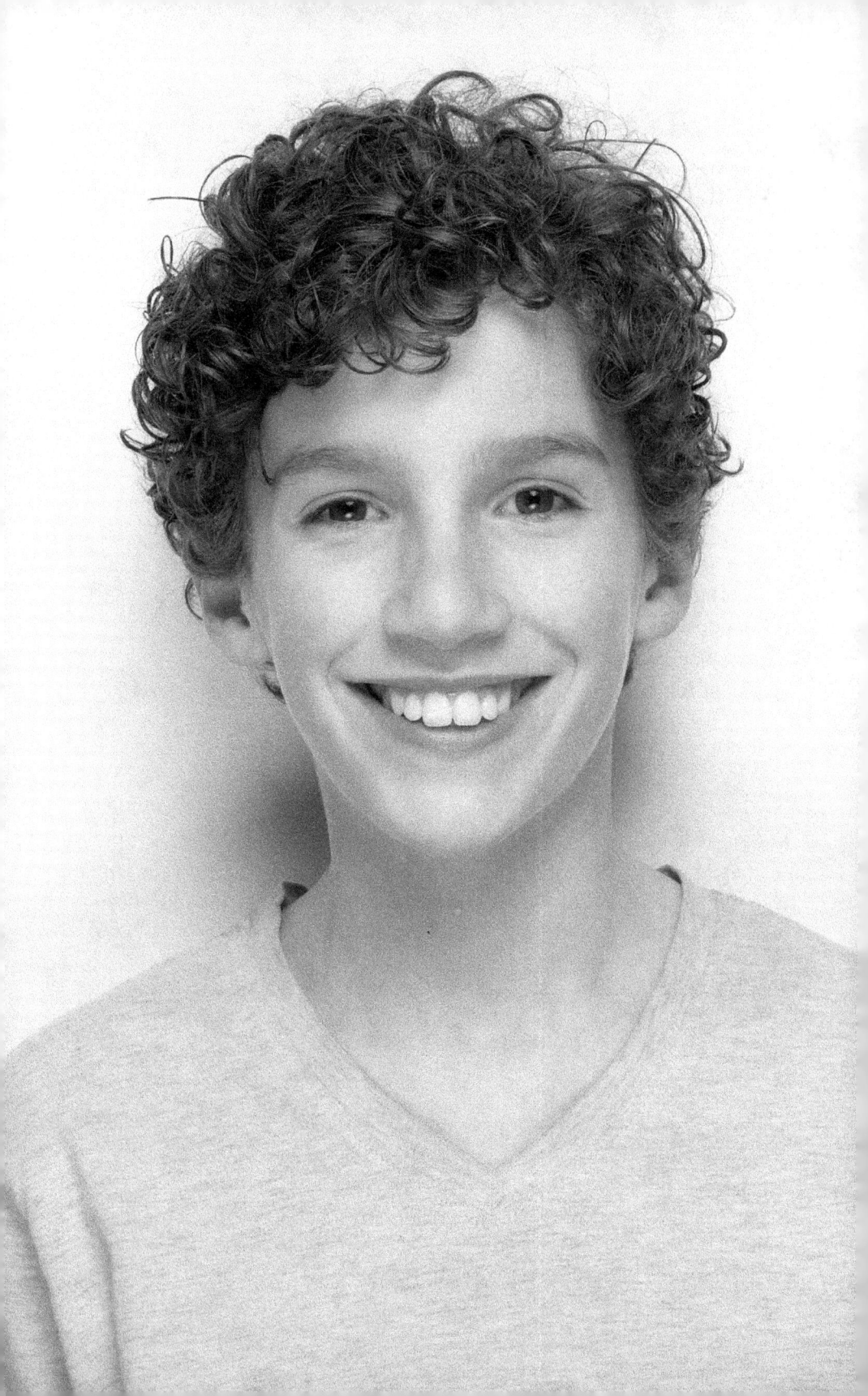

CHAPTER 7

What Are the Different Types of Braces Available?

Once you've found the "right" office, if your child is, indeed, ready for orthodontic care, one of the discussions you will have with your orthodontist is which type(s) of braces is/are right for your child.

If you're like most people, you probably are familiar with metal braces, but that is just one option that an orthodontist has and just one of the services he or she likely provides.

Here are four common tools that orthodontists use to move teeth and help patients reach their smile goals:

- Metal Braces
- Ceramic Braces – tooth-colored braces that blend in to natural tooth shades
- Lingual Braces – braces placed BEHIND your teeth
- Clear Aligners – such as Invisalign®, Clear Correct®, Elemetrix®, doctor-made, or any number of other brands

Metal Braces

Metal braces are the rock solid, gold standard of the orthodontic world...and the most popular treatment option for kids. Despite what the media may want you to think or believe, they aren't going away anytime soon, and kids absolutely love personalizing the braces with the different color options!

Today's metal braces are smaller, sleeker, and more polished than ever before. There are two main types. The first style requires an elastic o-shaped rubber band to hold the arch wire onto the bracket. These elastic ties often can easily collect plaque and bacteria, making it harder for patients to clean the teeth and gums.

The other type are called "self-ligating brackets", which means that the brackets do not need the little o-shaped rubber bands hold the wire in place. Instead there a clip or door built into the brace that does the job. This technology allows the wires to slide back and forth and often allows for longer time intervals between appointments, thus reducing the times that braces need "tightened". Since they don't have the o-shaped ties, it's harder to trap food and is easier to clean. With these type of braces, kids can still put color ties on, but they are strictly for "cosmetic" purposes!

Ceramic Braces

Ceramic braces "blend in" with the teeth and are much less noticeable than metal. (These are the type of braces actor Tom Cruise and singer Faith Hill had, by the way.) These are also a great choice for kids, especially if they are older teens or are self-conscious about having "metal" braces.

Older types of ceramic braces were brittle and required white or clear o-ties to hold the wire on to the braces. Patients would often complain that these ties would stain and look "yellow".

While some offices still use these, many are switching to self-ligating ceramic brackets. Just like their metal counterparts, they are very strong and have a door that holds the wire in place, instead of elastic ties. This is a huge advantage for aesthetic-conscious patients because self-ligating ceramic braces **will not stain** and are very durable!

The performance of today's ceramic braces is exactly the same as metal braces. Treatment is not compromised in any way and does not take any longer, as was the case in the past.

The cost of ceramic braces is usually more than the cost of metal braces, so many offices will pass along these supply costs to the patient as a part of their treatment fee, as add an additional charge to use ceramic an aesthetic "upgrade" over metal. Some offices, however, will charge the same for either metal or ceramic and just let the patient choose. Either way, be sure to ask your provider if there is a difference in cost to avoid any surprises!

Lingual Braces

Braces behind the teeth are the ONLY 100% INVISIBLE solution for straightening your teeth and are an awesome option for adults or kids where absolutely nothing can show on the front of the teeth.

Due to the custom fabrication of these braces, there will often be an increased cost to use them, but this is completely worth it for the patient who desires this solution. Additionally, because they are more challenging to work on, the appointments at your doctor's office may be more frequent and take a bit longer. Due to this added difficulty and increased appointment times, many offices will not offer lingual braces as a choice to patients. You will need to ask your orthodontist if this is an option, and, if not, they might be able to refer you to an office that does offer this treatment.

As much as it may seem like it, though, I have yet to have anyone tell me they are uncomfortable to wear or have interfered with their normal lifestyle in any way.   They do an awesome job!

Clear Aligner Therapy

For some kids, the thought of anything on the front or back of their teeth is not appealing, or their lifestyle necessitates that anything fixed to their teeth just won't work. Clear aligners (under various brand names such as Invisalign®, Clear Correct®, Elemetrix®, etc or those fabricated in your doctor's office) may then be a great choice. The advantage of clear aligners is that they are removable for cleaning, but the disadvantage is that they must be worn (and remembered to be worn 24/7 except meals and brushing) in order to work!

For the above options, ALL four ways will move teeth and ALL can work well when used appropriately. The conversation you will need to have with your orthodontist is figuring out where the teeth need to be and, THEN which method(s) can achieve those movements predictably and efficiently (not the other way around!) Once this is figured out, then you can choose with method you and your child would like to use.

In some cases, every option can be on the table, but in others, only one or two may work. Each person is different, and there is absolutely no one-size-fits-all solution. This is the critical discussion for you to have with your orthodontist in order to be realistic with the outcome and avoid frustration!

Call us at 484.730.1921 or go to www.coesmiles.com to schedule your own Customized Smile Analysis.

CHAPTER 8

Besides Braces, What Other Tools May My Orthodontist Use?

In addition to methods to align the teeth, your orthodontist may utilize other appliances to help align the underlying bones or change jaw position for your child prior to placing braces on the teeth. There are countless options available to orthodontists for these purposes, and too numerous to list all of them in this book. In my office, though, these are some of the most common I use, and I only use them because I have found them to have definitive, proven success in case after case when prescribed and used appropriately:

- Palate Expanders - to help match up the size of the upper jaw with the lower jaw as well as make space for the adult teeth
- Headgear – to help correct jaw alignment in growing patients (yes, it's still used and works amazingly well!)
- Bite Splints – to help relieve muscle and TMJ pain

Palate Expanders

An expander is an orthodontic appliance used to enlarge a small upper jaw on growing kids. Other than braces and retainers, this is the most common orthodontic treatment adjunct I use.

There are many variations of design, but the concept of use is identical. The expander is attached to either the teeth or directly to the upper jaw (in older kids) and the parent will use a key to activate it. Over the course of 4-6 weeks, depending on your child's expansion need, you will notice a dramatic change in the shape of your child's upper jaw, as well as more space for accommodating crowding teeth!

Parents often ask, since kids are growing, if an expander is needed or if it should wait. The reality is that, even with growth, a narrow upper jaw will always stay narrow with respect to the corresponding lower jaw. The only way to match things up is to intervene. I've yet to find any proven way in any orthodontic literature or my experience, other than using an expander, that accomplishes the same end result consistently.

For young kids, and even teenagers, expanders cause minimal discomfort, which is great. Yes, there is an adjustment period of a few days, but I have not encountered anyone who couldn't tolerate either the appliance or the activation (my own son included!). Best of all, I have definitely never had anyone tell me they weren't happy with the end result!

Your orthodontist will determine if you child would benefit from using an expander or not, and/or when it is indicated to do so. It's not a requirement for everyone to have one prior to braces, and definitely not a requirement for every young child to have one.

Be sure to ask your orthodontist how they determined if expansion is needed (or not) for your child. Some offices, unfortunately, will blanketly prescribe expansion to nearly everyone or, worse, not use expanders at all. Both scenarios, I feel, are equally dangerous and not in your child's best interest. Expansion treatment should be objectively based on a child's individual need, and is extremely successful when performed correctly in the correctly chosen case!

Headgear

"Headgear? Seriously? Orthodontists still use those things?" you may be asking.

Actually, yes. They work incredibly well and there's nothing available yet that compares to their effectiveness. While the premise of the appliance is similar, what has changed is how they are worn. Unlike in the 1960s and 1970s, they don't need to be worn all the time. Research has shown that, as long as they are worn when at home and during sleep hours, they will still work fine. With this protocol, no one even has to know your child has one! It's never to be worn outside of the house, when out with friends, or in other social situations.

There are two types of headgear and each differently affects the position of the jaws when they don't match up. One holds the upper jaw still while allowing the lower jaw to grow forward (in cases where there is a significant "overbite"). The other type helps the upper jaw move forward (when there is an "underbite").

Just like with expanders, headgear is not indicated for every child's case and only prescribed on a case-by-case need. However, unlike expanders, which are fixed in place, headgear is not so its effectiveness is dependent on it being used!

If determined to be appropriate for your child, your orthodontist will instruct you on proper usage.

Bite Splints

A bite splint is an appliance that, when properly adjusted, simulates an ideal bite in plastic. This is appropriate for people who have jaw or muscle pain or for patients who are known clenchers and grinders. While the appliances used for pain relief therapy are similar to those used for retention or nighttime wear, they differ in how they are prescribed for wear. Because the appliances used are adjusted to mimic an ideal bite and simulate an orthodontic outcome, the orthodontist is able to "test" a patient's response to orthodontic treatment to determine if changing the bite will have an effect on symptom relief. If these goals cannot be met, then definitive treatment of the bite with orthodontics may be contraindicated.

The purposes of bite splints are to relax the muscles, stabilize the jaw position, and provide the jaw joints (TMJs) with a stable environment to heal. While not especially common, it is surprising to see the number of kids who come in with jaw issues or pre-arthritis of their jaw joints, even with no overt pain.

Again, not every child will need or benefit from a bite split, but your orthodontist, through a through examination and looking at x-rays of the jaw joints can determine if a splint would be beneficial.

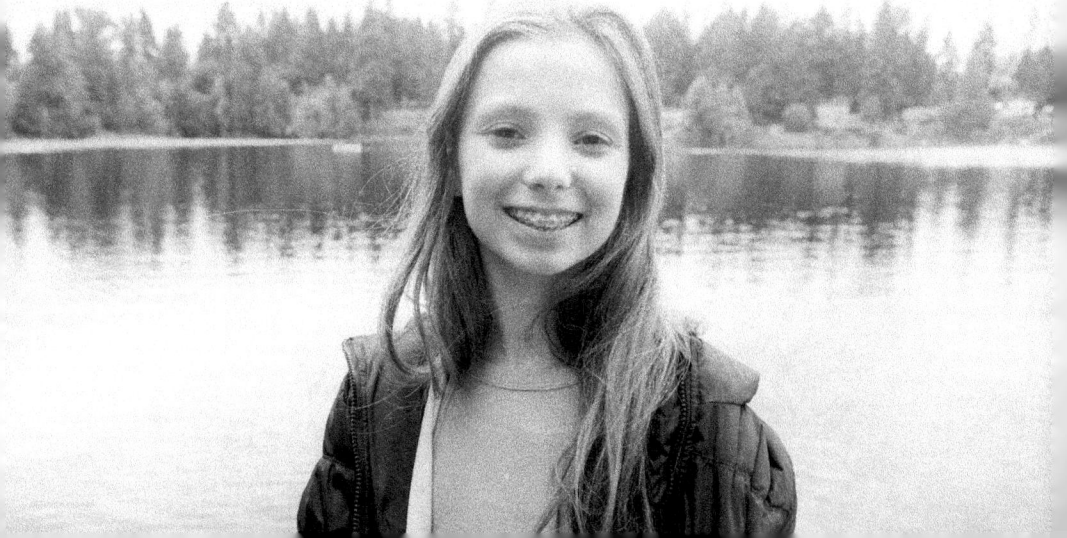

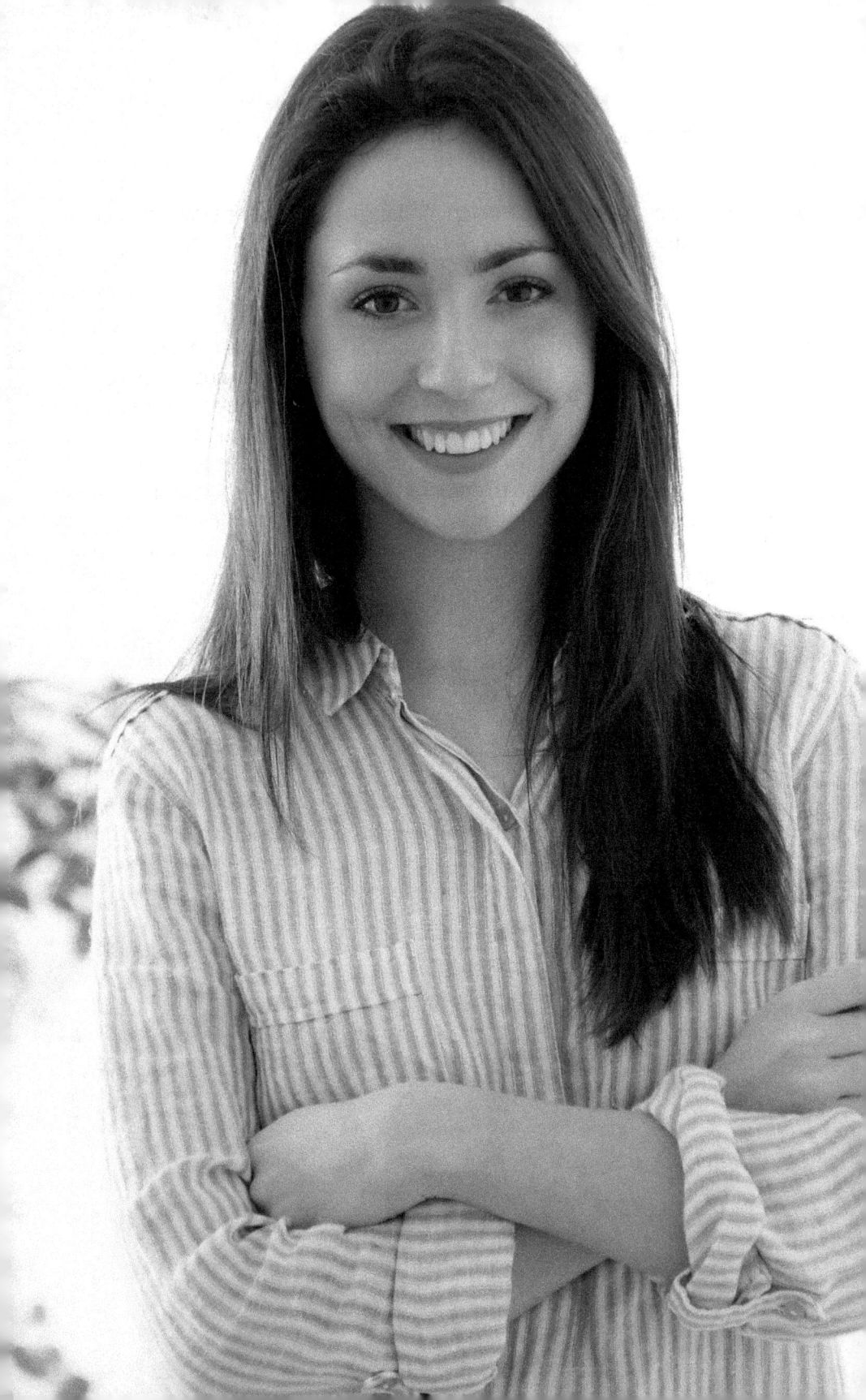

CHAPTER 9

Will My Child Need To Remove Any Adult Teeth?

Two of the phrases parents say a lot are, "I had teeth removed as a child, but I know that isn't done anymore, right?" or "I know technology has advanced since I had braces so I'm assuming my child won't need teeth removed to have braces, correct?"

In my experience, nothing strikes fear in a parent quicker than when they are told that their child will require adult teeth removed in order to have orthodontic treatment. Whether it is a fear of pain or discomfort for their child, a bad experience they had with tooth removal as a child, or just a sense that they "just don't want to" the thought of having to remove adult teeth makes them uneasy.

Understandable.

Here's the real scoop:

Truth: most orthodontists (including me!) would prefer NOT to remove adult teeth

Truth: orthodontic technology has advanced since the 1960s and 1970s to make treatment more comfortable and efficient, but no appliance or technology to date can overcome biology

Truth: when absolutely indicated to safely treat a child's bite, sometimes removal of adult teeth is indicated.

When I'm asked "What percent of patients in your practice do you recommend having adult teeth removed?" I always answer, "100% of those that would benefit from doing so, and 0% of those that wouldn't!" It's not sarcastic, just simply the truth!

My personal mission is to objectively help parents clearly understand why or why not removal of teeth is or isn't indicated. I help show how unattractive smiles or severe gum and bone loss in the future could result from NOT doing so (in cases where removal of teeth is indicated). Whoever you choose as your orthodontist should also have the same compassion and these same objectives.

Unfortunately, some orthodontists play into this innate parental "fear" of removing adult teeth and will claim they NEVER remove teeth, say that removal of adult teeth is "old-fashioned" treatment, or claim that the types of braces/techniques they use are "special" and avoid having to remove teeth. Additionally, one of the latest scare tactics on the internet suggests that removing teeth as will lead to any one of a number of chronic conditions as an adult, including sleep apnea*.

All these statements are not only false, but are simply marketing pitches from companies and orthodontists so their businesses can financially benefit, regardless for any actual benefit to your child. These sentiments are also extremely dangerous and irresponsible, as this means the orthodontist is looking at cramming all the teeth in as the sole objective...without understanding the role of the other structures of your child's face and bite play as a part of the big picture!

> Be very wary of any orthodontist that claims they NEVER remove any adult teeth or, worse, say that the types of braces/ techniques they use avoid people having to remove teeth. This is simply not statistically or biologically possible for everyone!

As stated previously, my preference, just like most orthodontists, would be to NOT have to remove teeth. However, as a realist looking out for every child's best long-term interest, sometimes it's beneficial, and I have to keep all options on the table!

I only suggest tooth removal when all other methods to avoid doing so are exhausted, and when it's objectively in your child's best interest. The orthodontist you ultimately choose for your family should also feel the same way!

---

*In cases where the orthodontist does not respect or diagnose all parts of a patient's chewing system and airway, this absolutely could occur. However, as a standalone statement there is no scientific evidence to prove this. It is simply a marketing pitch. If you are concerned about this or anything you may have heard or read, be sure your orthodontist helps you understand how breathing issues with respect to tooth position will affect your child.

The bottom-line is that you, as a parent, have to feel comfortable and clearly know the reasons why tooth removal is or is not indicated. Your orthodontist should adequately, and ideally objectively, explain why or why not your child would benefit from either decision and you should feel comfortable with their recommendation. If you do not, by all means then you SHOULD seek a second opinion!

Call us at 484.730.1921 or go to www.coesmiles.com to schedule your own Customized Smile Analysis.

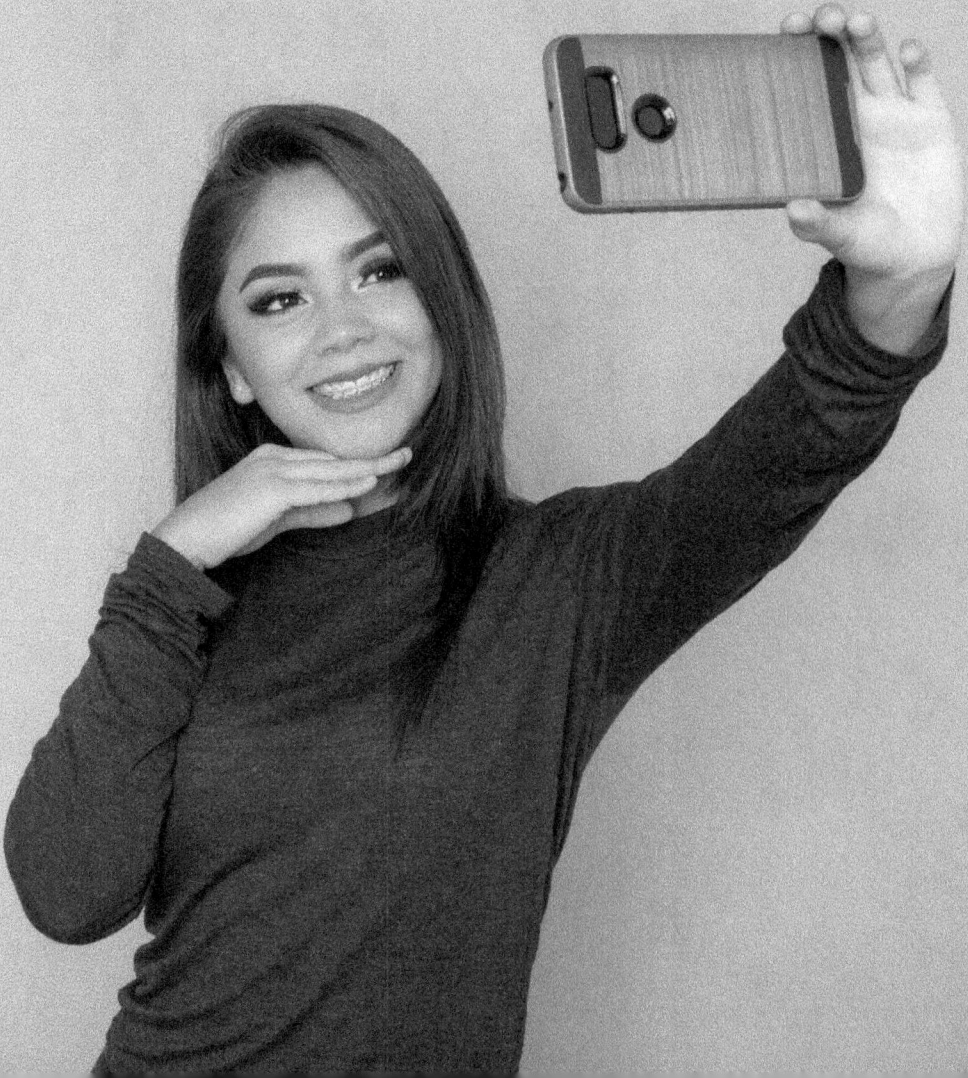

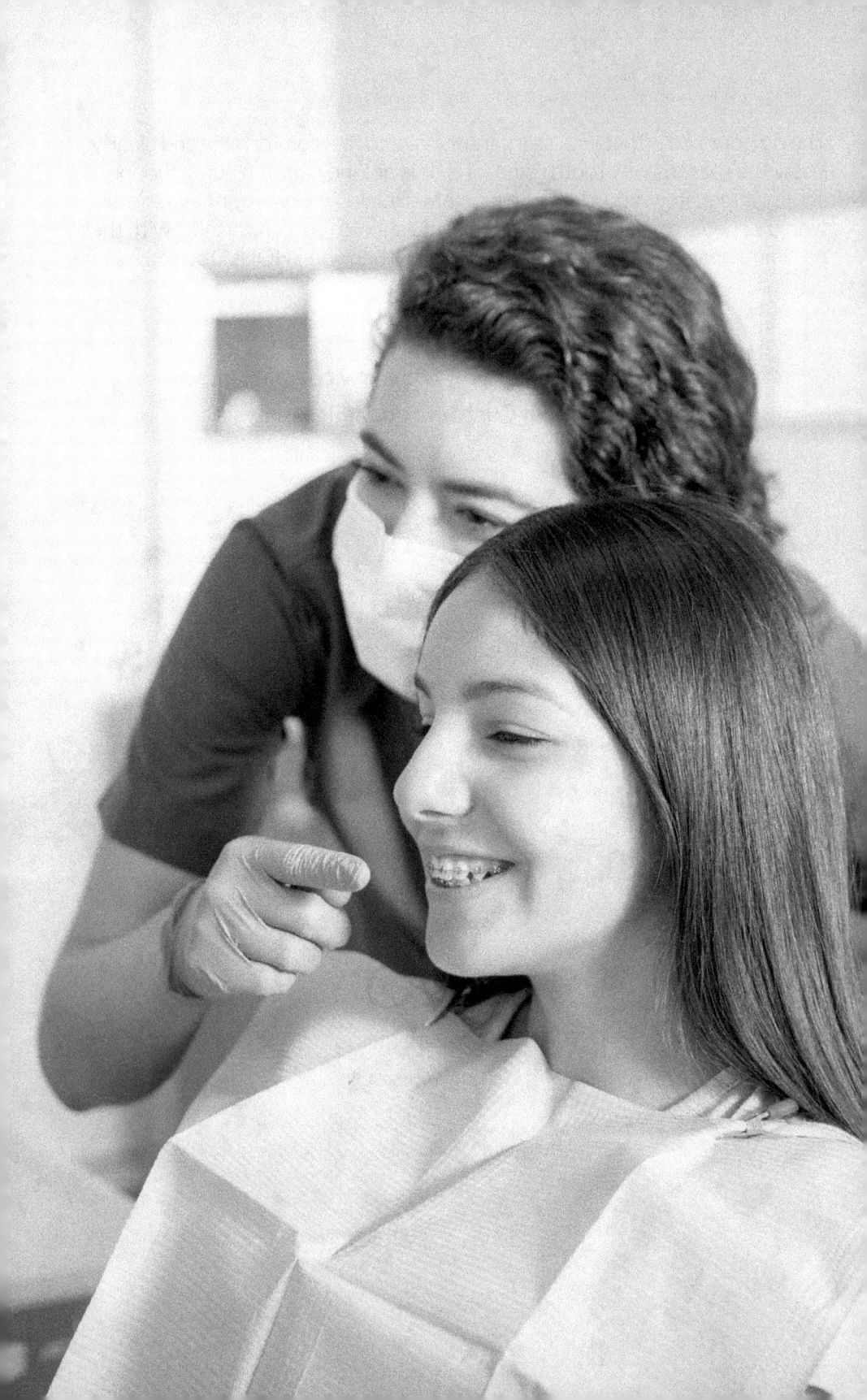

CHAPTER 10

Fitting Orthodontic Treatment Into Your Family's Budget

As a parent in the communities, I serve, I know life is crazy busy and getting reliable, honest information quickly can be tough. I hope this book has been helpful so far with understanding orthodontic treatment. However, on the non-treatment side, I've found that many questions come up with how to finance orthodontic treatment and that many families are just as confused here as well!

I've been fortunate to have thousands of families trust the conservative approach I use to determine what treatment, if any at all, is appropriate to give their kids a winning smile, how it can fit into their busy schedules, and... how to make it easily affordable! My office prides itself in personalizing the braces experience as well as customizing the financing to fit into anyone's budget, so I want to empower other parents and share this information as they embark on their own orthodontic journey.

With this chapter you will learn how to:

- Pre-plan a budget to alleviate financial stress
- Use FSA/HSA to maximize your tax deductions and offset braces
- Recognize 6 common misconceptions about dental "insurance"

Finding a Budget That Works For YOU!

My goal is always to make 100% sure finances don't stand in the way of getting a great smile and allowing our patients' lives to shine! However, we always hear that one of the biggest concerns families have with starting orthodontic treatment at other offices is fitting it into their monthly budget.

This is where your orthodontist needs your help! You will learn through reading this chapter that there is typically a portion of orthodontic treatment that will not be covered by dental insurance benefits or other means. Therefore, you will need figure out a way to accommodate the balance, either by paying it in full or breaking it down into installments to minimize the impact to your family's budget.

As a very, very, very rough ballpark figure, the average total orthodontic treatment cost for full adolescent braces is typically between $5000-7000. What that fee includes will vary among offices, so be sure to ask...as it's often not apples to apples. Some offices are all-inclusive. Some offices blatantly advertise "super-cheap" base fees, but then have hidden or add-on fees for various portions of treatment, fine-print terms that you don't find out until later, or place restrictions on what the "cheap" fee includes.

Just like with most things in life, you get what you pay for, so don't be lured in by a seemingly "low" price without doing your homework. There's often a catch! You should not have to play detective with orthodontic treatment costs for your family. Great questions to ask are:

- Are retainers included?
- What happens if my child breaks or loses a retainer?
- Is there a charge for broken appliances?
- Is there a charge for after-hours visits?
- Are there extra charges if treatment takes longer than anticipated?
- Are there additional charges for adjunctive appliances (such as expanders, Invisalign®, etc.)

The most honest offices will be completely transparent and forthright with both fees charged and benefits received. You deserve nothing less, and definitely no funny business with this regard!

Understanding Dental Benefits and Payment Plans

If you are fortunate to have dental benefits (aka dental "insurance"), they will often assist anywhere between $1000-2000 of this cost, with the remaining portion being your responsibility. With an average plan of $1500 of benefit, this means the portion you are responsible for (in an average case fee of $5000-7000) will be between ~$3500-5500.

One thing that can really help the orthodontic process go smoothly is to recognize there will be out of pocket costs that you can either pay-in-full (often with a "thank you" discount) or split up into a downpayment and monthly payments.

We see a common barrier to moving forward with treatment for your child is the parent who brings the child in for the initial consultation, goes through the entire process to figure out treatment needs, agrees to the treatment plan, is ready to start, but then needs to speak with other spouse about payment options.

> To minimize delays, you should have a discussion with your spouse about what ballpark downpayment and/or range of monthly payment you would feel comfortable with BEFORE you even come into the office!

For some families, this could be $1500 down, $1000 down, or $250 down, with monthly payments of $500/month, $300/month, $150/month, or $100/month. It does not matter what your comfortable downpayment or monthly number is (a great smile can cost even less than your cell phone bill per month!) and every family's budget is different. However, you need make sure you communicate with your orthodontic team what range works for you, and then they should be able to do everything possible to work within it to help you get the smile you want!

Therefore, if you know you are ready to proceed with treatment, speaking with your spouse or working through your monthly finances prior to visiting your orthodontist's office will help them tailor a plan that fits your needs and gets your child smiling as easily as possible!

Take Advantage of Flex Spending/Health Savings Accounts (FSA/HSA)!

Flex Spending Accounts (FSA) or Health Savings Accounts (HSA) set up through your employer are fantastic ways to offset the costs of orthodontic treatment as well as help you reduce your tax burden for the year. They can be combined with insurance benefits and should be utilized to the fullest extent possible when they are available for your family! Many programs allow for significant pre-tax contributions of $1000, $2500, or even $5000, as long as you plan in advance. Be sure to talk to your Human Resources representative or visit www.healthcare.gov for more information.

Since the FSA/HSA can be used for any portion of orthodontic treatment, you need to take advantage of this to get the added tax benefit. However, the one catch with FSAs is that you have to use any money that is placed in this account by the year-end, or you LOSE it. Yes, that's terrible, but unfortunately, it's the law and there is no way to pull money out for non-medical needs. Funds placed in HSA accounts can rollover to the following year and are much more flexible, so be sure you know which type of savings plan you have!

The bottom line is:

- **FSA/HSA plans give significant tax savings and are fantastic ways to offset orthodontic costs**
- **Plan strategically to make sure you have available funds to cover your orthodontic expenses**
- **Don't over-fund the account if you don't think you'll need it or your child isn't ready to start**
- **You only have one chance per year to enroll, so pre-planning is critical**

Your orthodontist can help you determine both if orthodontic treatment is going to be indicated to start in the upcoming year, as well as help you determine how you should contribute to your plan.

If you have a family accountant, you may want to consult with him about your HSA or FSA to ensure your contributions are indeed deductible.

Finally, be aware of "family status changes" allowed by your plan that may enable you to change the amount being moved pre-tax from your paychecks to your account anytime during the year rather than just once at the first of the year—so you could bump up the amount in months before the first orthodontic treatment.

Six Little Known Facts About Insurance!

If you are fortunate to have a dental benefits plan through your employer or on your own (also known as dental "insurance") this is a great way to help offset orthodontic costs! Dental benefits policies are separate from any medical benefits you may have and both are separate policies with different terms of coverage. Orthodontists cannot file claims for treatment under medical insurance, nor are there provisions to do so.

Unlike medical insurance, dental benefits for orthodontics are not "insurance" in the sense that it protects you from financial hardship in the event of a catastrophe. Instead of covering you for an unanticipated prolonged medical illness, home loss from fire, or similar circumstances, orthodontic dental benefits are simply an amount of money that the insurance company will provide for you to offset costs of orthodontic treatment if they are a part of your policy. Typically this amount ranges from $1000-2000, depending on the policy you or your employer have chosen for your family.

I find that many patients are not aware of how dental benefits work, and it definitely can be confusing! However, it's important for you to check out your own plan so there are no surprises and you can become better informed when choosing coverage for your family!

Here are six common misunderstandings I hear on a daily basis from families, so I hope this helps you better understand your policy!

1. Orthodontic benefits are a lifetime amount per person

Once they are used, provided you keep the same policy, no additional benefit remains and it does not reset on a yearly basis or get refreshed. Your yearly premium that you pay for the dental policy will remain the same even after the orthodontic benefit is used.

2. Most plans will set limits on coverage

Take a look at your plan carefully! Using language, such as 50% coverage up to $1500 means that they will cover orthodontic treatment at 50% of the submitted fee, but only reimburse a maximum of $1500, with the balance to be out-of-pocket. Let's consider a few examples:

If the total cost of treatment is $6000, the company will provide the full $1500 towards offsetting this cost (50% of $6000 is $3000, and they will provide the full $1500 of coverage. Then the remaining $4500 will be out-of-pocket).

However, if the total cost of treatment is $2000, the company will only provide $1000 of coverage (because this is 50% of the treatment fee, with the other $1000 being out-of-pocket). $500 of benefit will then remain for another procedure on another date.

It's important to know your limits of coverage as well as any benefits that remain. Coverage is not specific to one office or a provider, so if you move and have to switch providers but keep the same policy, your limits do not reset!

3. Many dental assistance programs for children require a pre-qualification to actually use the benefits you are paying for!

This qualification is a subjective evaluation by an insurance company employee (who has never actually seen your child) to determine if your child "qualifies" to even use the benefits you've paid for. This is based on a "score" with point values given to various aspects of the bite.

Many times, these programs will say the child's dental issues are not severe enough or "medically necessary" so they will not provide coverage. **THIS DOES NOT MEAN YOUR CHILD WOULDN'T BENEFIT FROM ORTHODONTIC TREATMENT**. It only means the program will not contribute to offsetting the costs, even though you may have paid for the benefit.

This is a common issue that frustrates many parents, and understandably so, but this decision is ultimately up to the company providing the benefits and the evaluator who has never actually seen your child, NOT you or your child's orthodontic provider.

While it is unfortunate that coverage might be denied, the bonus is that you are now free to see whatever provider you choose, not just the ones limited to the assistance program!

I have not seen this issue arise with a PPO (preferred provider organization) benefits policy, where you are free to use your benefit regardless of provider or severity, but the "rules" are always subject to change!

4. Many dental benefit plans have exclusions for "adult" orthodontic treatment

Often companies provide the benefit for immediate family members (with maximum age limits up to 19 or 25), but not for "adults". If you DO have adult orthodontic benefits included as part of your benefits package, consider yourself very lucky and be sure to take advantage of using them if your "child" is over 18!

5. Dental benefits are not a requirement to begin orthodontic treatment

Many families who do not have dental benefits say they do not want to start orthodontic treatment until they get them. However, it is important to evaluate the true costs of doing so and often it might be more economical to NOT get dental benefits for only orthodontic reasons.

The orthodontic benefit is usually not provided in one lump sum, but is broken down into installments over the course of treatment. In order to get the full amount of the orthodontic benefit, you have to keep the policy active the entire time. By the time you are finished with treatment, many times the premiums paid over multiple years will be close to or even exceed the benefit received, so no savings was realized.

Be sure to check on this and do the math to see if the situation makes sense for your family!

6. Your policy must remain active throughout orthodontic treatment

If you change jobs or your dental benefits policy is cancelled, any remaining portion of the benefit will typically become your out-of-pocket responsibility. So, if your plan provides $1500 of coverage that is broken down into even installments over a two-year orthodontic plan, but you change jobs after 1 year, the remaining $750 becomes your responsibility.

Many times these differences can be re-submitted to the new dental benefits company, but be aware that sometimes they will not be approved for work that is "in progress".

While every dental benefits plan is different, your orthodontic office's team members are experts with helping you maximize your dental benefits and helping sort through any confusion. They should always be available to answer any questions and help you understand the policy that you or your employer has chosen for your family!

> **Call us at 484.730.1921 or go to www.coesmiles.com to schedule your own Customized Smile Analysis.**

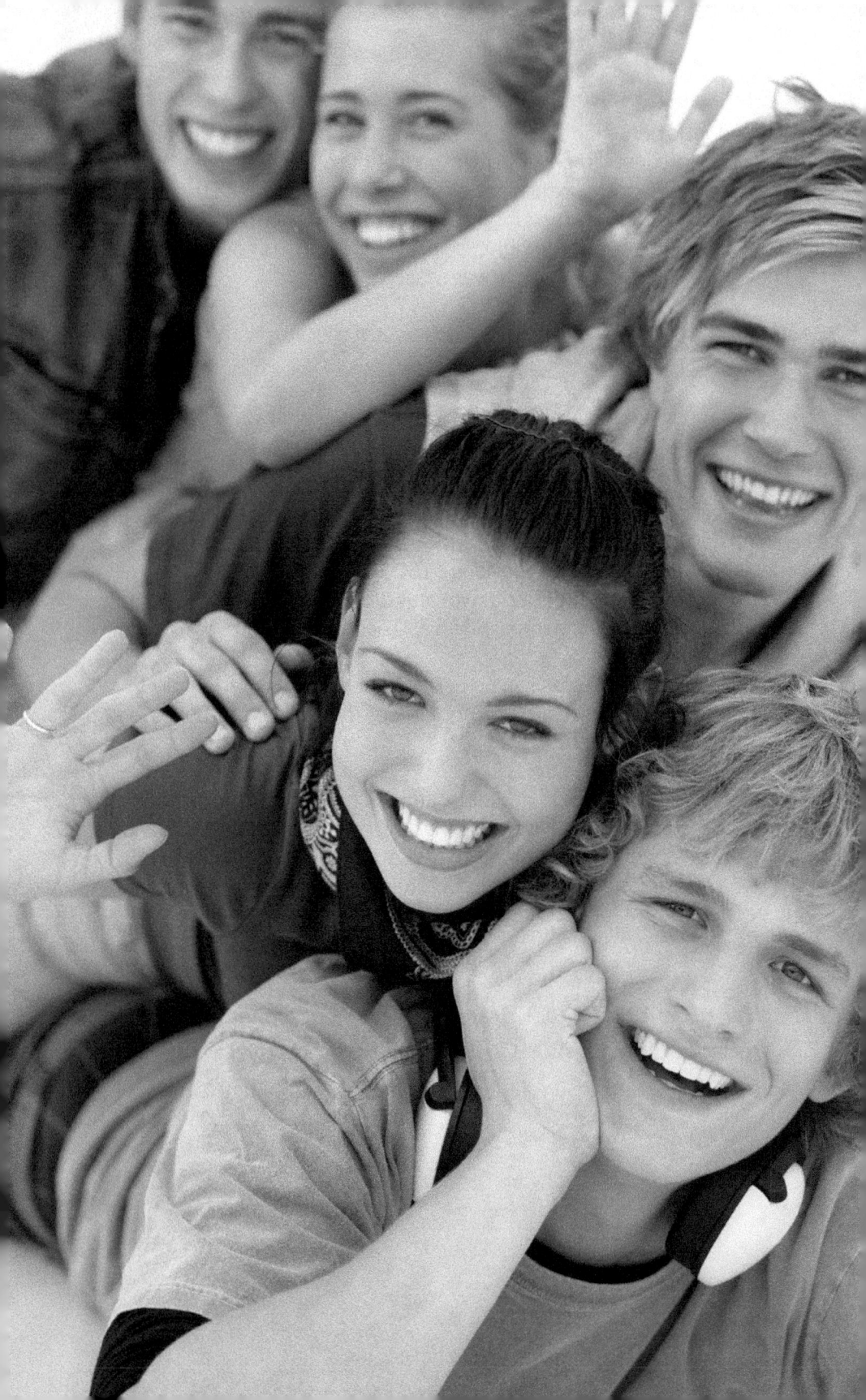

CHAPTER 11

Life with Braces!

Remember, today's orthodontic care is far more advanced, more sophisticated, and more patient-centered than any prior generation has experienced.

Living with braces is not going to be anywhere near as difficult as you might imagine and most treatment proceeds pretty uneventfully and fits seamlessly in patient's lives.

Let's look at a few specific concerns.

Brushing and Hygiene

Modern orthodontic appliances, whether they are metal, ceramic, or removable, are all actually made to facilitate easy brushing. You can use either an electric or a manual toothbrush. It does not matter what type, as long as it is USED!

Here are some simple tips you can share with your child for the best results when brushing with braces on:

- Brush your teeth with a soft or medium nylon toothbrush after you eat and before bed.
- Brush, rinse, and look; if you find any areas that are not clean, brush them again.
- Brush your gums as you brush your teeth (massage and stimulate).
- Take extra care in the area between the gums and the braces, because food caught and left there can cause swollen gums, cavities, discomfort, and permanent teeth stains.
- Replace your old toothbrush when it gets worn out.
- Continue regular visits to your family dentist for checkups and cleanings throughout your orthodontic treatment – you MUST do this!

Depending on the age of your child, you, the parent, may need to supervise the first few brushings with the braces in place. It should be painless, simple, and routine.

If the gums get red, puffy, or bleed, this is unlikely due to the appliances. In ultra-rare cases, some patients react to the material in the wires, but this is not commonplace. Instead, this occurs when plaque and old food are not adequately brushed away, especially around the gumlines. The body reacts, and the gums get tender, which makes brushing the area tough, which causes more food to accumulate, which causes further swelling, and the cycle continues.

THEREFORE, YOU MUST BRUSH NOT ONLY THE BRACES AND TEETH, BUT ALSO THE GUMLINE!!!

In cases of poor hygiene, your orthodontist may remove the wires until the swelling goes down, which will ultimately delay treatment and prolong how long you have to wear braces. In severe cases, appliances may even be removed, often without a refund.

Foods To Avoid

After your child's braces have been placed, the teeth are often "tender" and sensitive for 3-10 days. During these few days, softer foods are recommended: soups, macaroni, spaghetti, eggs, fish, or yogurt. As needed, Tylenol or Advil are more than adequate in relieving any discomfort, taken an hour or so before eating.

For the entire duration of the braces being in place, stay away from hard, sticky, sugary foods that can damage braces and may lengthen the time they have to be worn and require extra office visits.

1. Hard foods: Ice, nuts, popcorn (has hard kernels inside), peanut brittle, rock candy, whole apples and carrots (unless cut into bite sized pieces), corn on the cob, hard pretzels, hard rolls, hard taco shells. Note: no chewing on pencils or pens.

2. Sticky foods: Starbursts, caramel, bubble gum, taffy, and sticky rolls.

3. Chewy foods: Pizza crust, bagels, beef jerky, gummy bears.

4. Super-sugary drinks: Soda, excessive juices, energy drinks.

Your orthodontist will speak about this with your son or daughter, but you will have to reinforce this general list at home. Bottom line, if you think it is too hard, sticky, chewy, or sweet it probably is. Use good judgment. Most kids get it, though, and are pretty responsible when it comes to watching what they eat.

Emergencies/Repairs/Comfort Visits

One great thing about orthodontic treatment is that there are rarely any "true emergencies". Yes, there may be some inconveniences, but life-threatening concerns are almost unheard of.

Common issues that arise, such as poking wires or loose braces that need repaired are NOT, I repeat, NOT emergencies. These comfort and repair issues can easily be remedied with information found on your orthodontist's website or on the internet. However, you will want to call your orthodontist's office so they can see you to fix them as soon as possible.

If you have an injury to the face (such as getting hit with a ball) and your teeth are loose, your mouth is bleeding, or you suspect broken bones, this needs attention immediately! Call you orthodontist's office for instructions on how to proceed, as well as your family dentist's office, and get to the emergency room to be checked out!

Vacations/Trips

If anything should happen while you are on vacation or away from home, your orthodontist can help guide you with advice, or even arrange to have you see a local colleague wherever you may be! We are all here to help and want to see your child brace-free and smiling as soon as possible!

Sports and Musical Instruments

Yes, your child can participate in all sports and play all musical instruments during treatment. Every orthodontic office I am aware of has patients that are involved in football, soccer, softball, trumpet, saxophone, piano, singing, dancing, and acting and have braces on their teeth. Your child can definitely do all of them and I'm not aware of any budding careers that were cut short while getting a better smile!

For all sports, I recommend a mouthguard be worn to help prevent against concussions and inadvertent trauma to the teeth. Your orthodontist can help recommend a style they prefer.

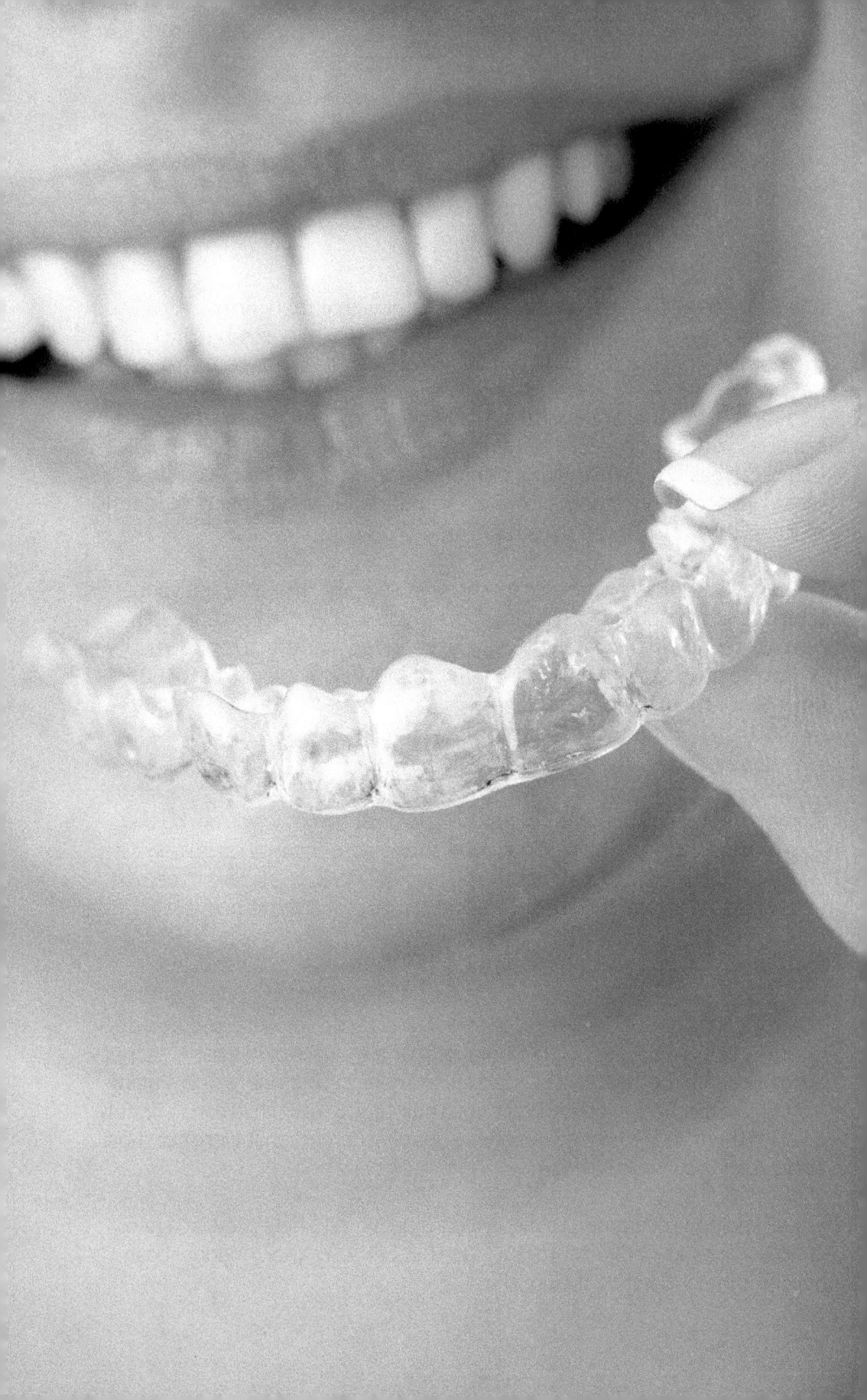

CHAPTER 12

Life After Braces!

So, your child's braces are off and they're ready to live a life full of confidence and good oral health. They may think, I'm free! I'm free! Well, not quite yet.

The selection of the right braces, the expert orthodontist, and the compliance of the patient with instructions gets us about three-fourths of the way to where we want to be: a well-aligned, as-perfect-as-possible, healthy smile for life.

But after braces, there are retainers.

When the braces are removed, teeth can still shift if not helped through a period of adjustment, to settle in. Retainers gently but purposefully remind the teeth to stay straight during this adjustment period.

Years ago, clinicians believed that once teeth were straightened by braces, they would simply stay that way forever. New science says otherwise. In fact, teeth position shifting as we age is to be expected. Teeth naturally shift to the middle and crowd. So, retainers are actually extremely important in maintaining the new smile from braces.

There are many different styles available for retainers and all serve a different purpose. However, they are all customized specifically to your mouth, your bite, and your needs. Your orthodontist will choose what is appropriate for you!

Additionally, every orthodontist has their own protocol and instructions for how to properly wear and care for your retainers. Your job is to follow it, keep your retainers in good shape, and enjoy your great smile for life!

So, the answer for the common question, "How long do I have to wear my retainers?" is..."as long as you want your teeth to remain straight".

> **Call us at 484.730.1921 or go to www.coesmiles.com to schedule your own Customized Smile Analysis.**

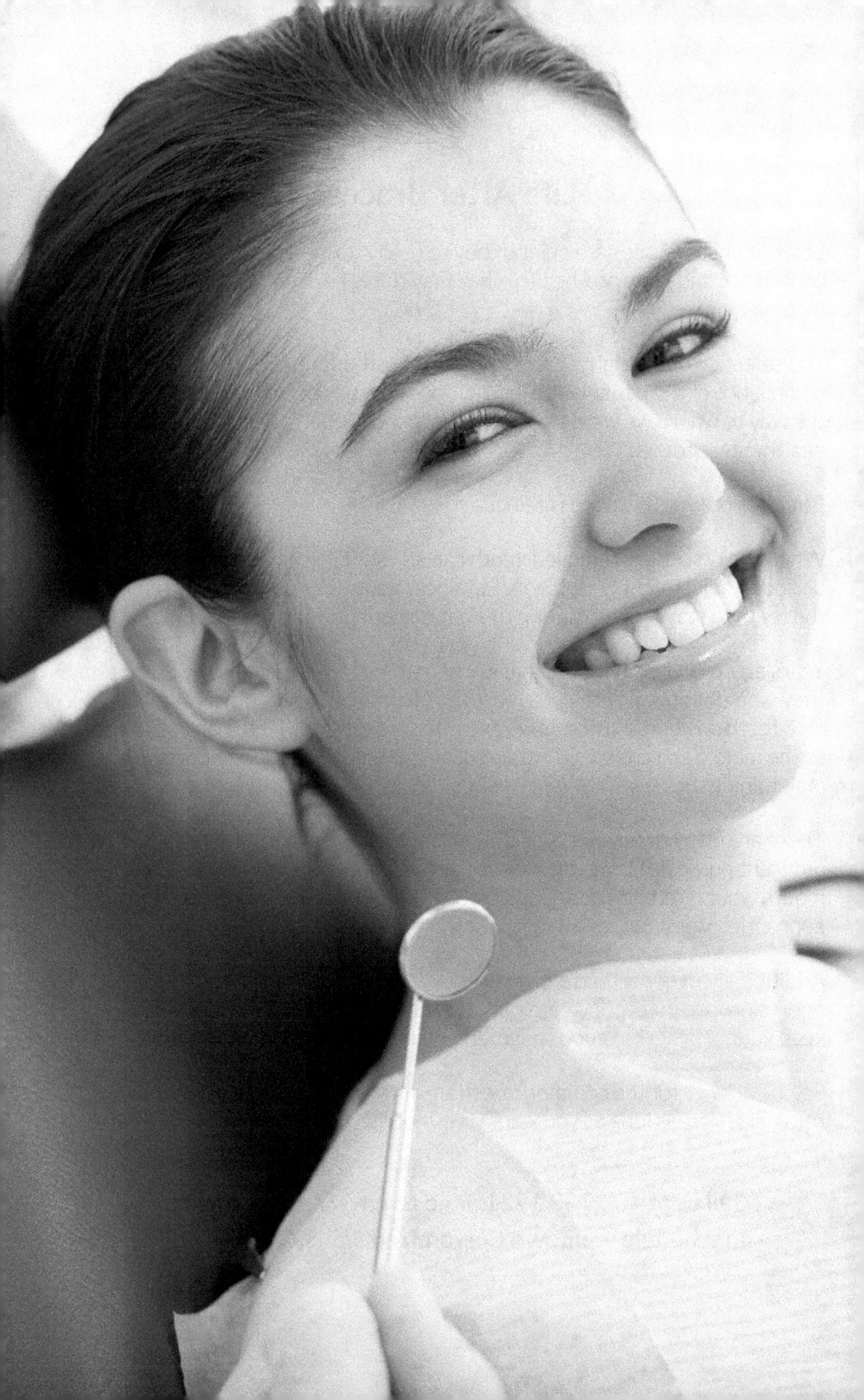

CHAPTER 13

LET'S CELEBRATE!

I love seeing patients celebrate getting their braces off. There are so many ways your child can celebrate, but here are a few options your child may want to consider:

- **Throw a party.** Did anyone ever need an excuse to have a party? Well here's one for sure! Throwing a "braces are off" party is a great way to celebrate. Invite friends over, put out the foods that they've been longing for, and enjoy showing off those new straight teeth.

- **Plan a photo shoot.** Your child deserves to show the world his new beautiful smile! Plan a photo shoot, so he can be one-on-one with a photographer and put his best smile forward. He'll get some great shots and can show all his friends on social media his new look.

- **Go caramel.** Now is the time your child can sink his teeth into something like a caramel apple. No more avoiding the caramel and cutting the apple into bite-sized pieces. Nope, he can actually eat a full caramel apple, right off the stick! He can get one at the mall or a carnival or even make them himself. Either way, he'll love being able to bite into that sticky gooey sweetness worry free!

- **Break out the selfie stick.** Go nuts. Post brace-free pictures on Facebook, Instagram, Snapchat, or whatever your favorite social media site is! Give your orthodontist and family shout-outs for helping you get through this awesome journey!

Of course, nobody can celebrate finishing unless they get started. There really is no time like the present to do so!

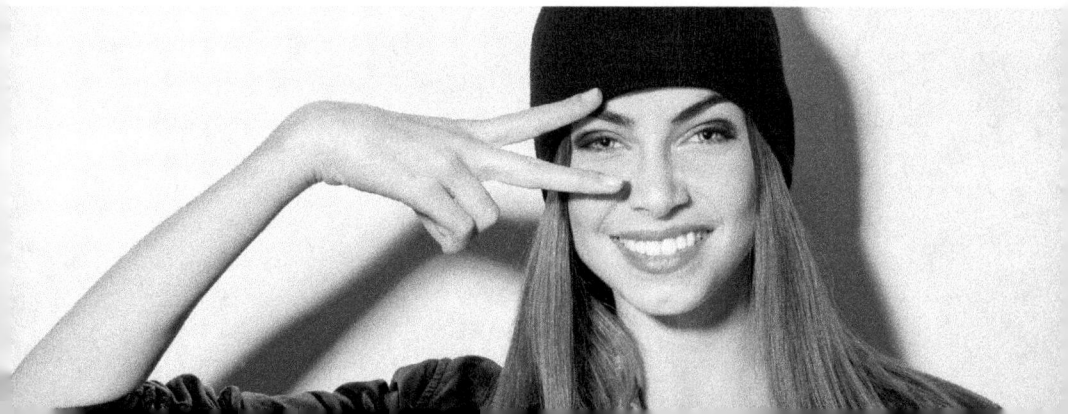

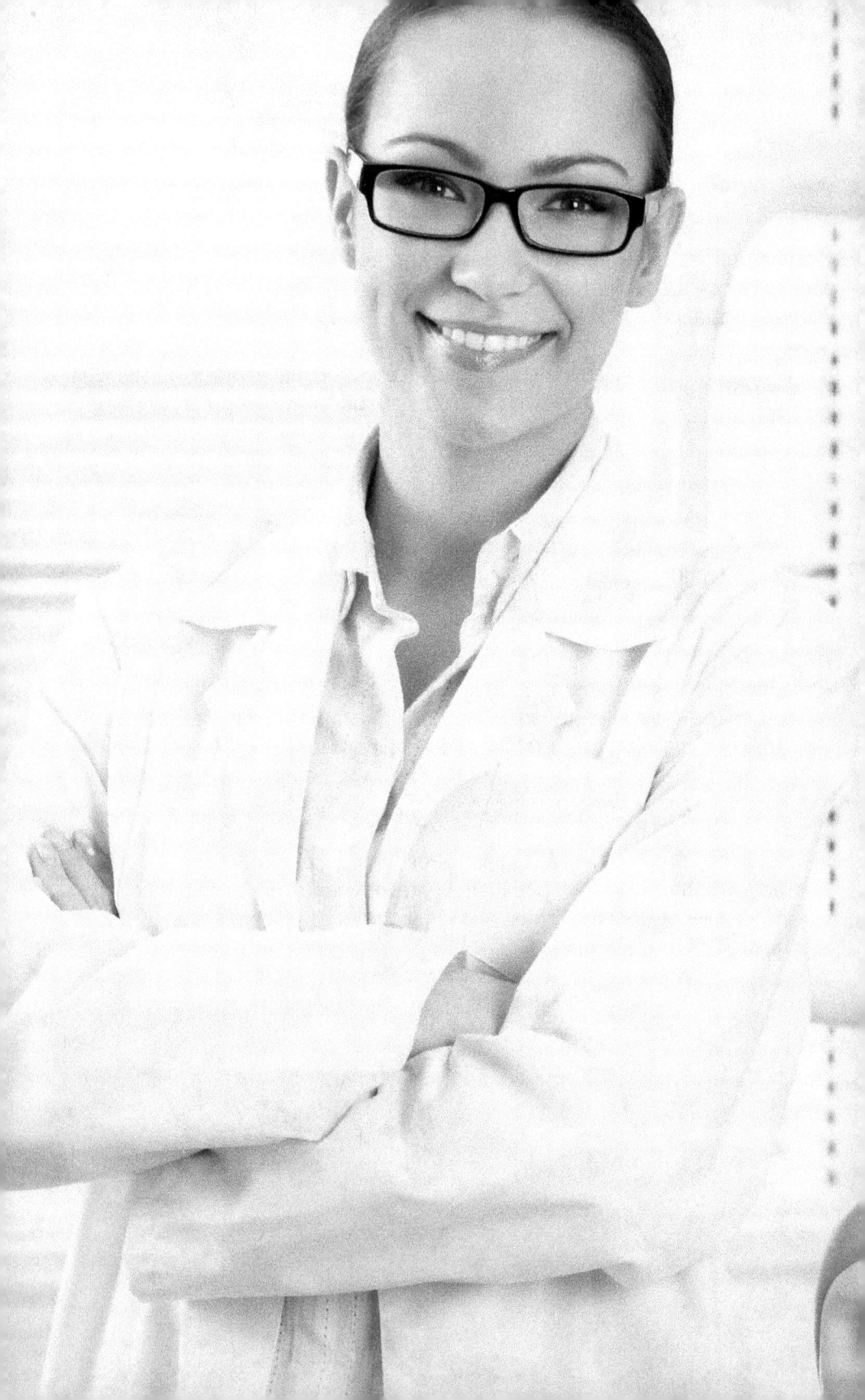

CHAPTER 14

What About *My* Smile?

Mom and Dad, you read this book and are now ready to take on the ortho world for your kids, right? However, some of the words may have sparked some thoughts in your mind. You've looked in the mirror, saw your crooked teeth, and always thought about doing something about it but never did. You now think you're too old, and nothing can be done. Both thoughts are false and you're actually in luck.

Adult orthodontic treatment is super common today, and with many of the non-metal options described in the previous chapter, you can get also get a great smile discreetly and easily.

You may be surprised that a significant portion of your child's orthodontic office actually IS adults in their 30s, 40s, 50s, or 60s. When you go to the office at 3:45 PM in the afternoon, it may just look like kids, but often the "adults" prefer to come in the morning or around lunchtime, so you just don't see them.

Adults are not "big kids" and have to be treated a bit differently, but as long as your teeth and gums are healthy, getting a great smile should be no problem!

The only way to know what the options are is with a complete, expert orthodontic exam. Talk to your child's orthodontist about your options and if they take adult patients. If so, you may be able to go from an embarrassing smile you often hide to a beautiful smile you love – and do it at the same time as your child – for an awesome parent/child bonding experience!

Call us at 484.730.1921 or go to www.coesmiles.com to schedule your own Customized Smile Analysis.

10 FREQUENTLY ASKED QUESTIONS (JUST THE FAQ'S, MA'AM)

FAQ #1: "Shouldn't I wait until all permanent teeth come in before my child sees an orthodontist for their first visit?"

Definitely not! The American Association of Orthodontists recommends children should have their first orthodontic evaluation at age 7. I agree. Seeing someone at this age provides a nice baseline for their jaw structure and you can get information on what to expect over the next 4-5 years. Furthermore, there are many subtle factors to proper growth and development that are best corrected when the bones are easily moldable. If indicated, early treatment can help alleviate many developmental problems or difficulties with treatment that would ensue if treatment is delayed.

FAQ #2: "Do permanent teeth always have to be removed for orthodontic treatment?"

Absolutely not! While I would like to say that this isn't needed anymore and orthodontists never recommend removal of permanent teeth, this would not be truthful. In certain cases it is necessary to remove adult teeth to meet smile goals and maintain gum and bone health for patients. If removal of adult teeth are indicated for providing an optimal result, the rationale for doing so should be objectively determined and reviewed in detail with the patient!

FAQ #3: "My neighbor's son/daughter has braces and he/she is only 8 years old. I thought this was just for teenagers. Are orthodontists doing braces sooner now?"

Without knowing the definite reasons, I cannot specify or comment on the reasons you may see a young child in treatment. However, as a rough answer, no, they aren't, but orthodontists are more aware of the benefits that interceping developmental issues has on a child's overall development. Treatment at an early age usually deals with working on the underlying bones, not the teeth (although many orthodontists do align the teeth at the same time). Also, this treatment does not substitute for "braces" later in life. It can be thought of in this way: when indicated, treatment when young is done to set up the jaws properly, then "braces" later in life focuses on aligning and correcting the teeth and bite.

FAQ #4: "If my child has orthodontic treatment early, does this mean they won't need braces when the permanent teeth are all in?"

In most instances, the answer is "no". As stated previously, "early treatment" or "Phase 1" is generally done to set up the foundation of the jaws, assist growth and development, and to help guide the eruption of the permanent teeth. Once the jaws are the optimal size and the permanent teeth have come in, moving teeth around becomes very routine and leads to a more predictable outcome. Some kids will be lucky and all of their adult teeth will come in perfectly, but usually they still will benefit from braces to clean up some crowding, close a few spaces, and ultimately get the bite perfect.

FAQ #5: "What is your price for braces? Can you quote a price over the phone or just look in my mouth and be able to tell me the cost?"

This question is equivalent to you calling your car dealership without any details of the problem and saying, "My car won't start. How much will you charge to fix it?" Without doing a proper examination, diagnostic workup, and through analysis of your child's specific case, it's impossible to quote an exact fee or give you a definitive treatment plan. Therefore, once your orthodontist determines your child's needs, then they can discuss any associated costs.

FAQ #6: "Is tightening braces painful for my child?"

This is a common misconception because braces are not "tightened". At the adjustment visits, the thickness and shape of the wire are changed in order to guide the teeth into the proper positions. While this does lead to mild soreness (especially on the front teeth) for a few days following appointments, the pressure applied is gradual and any discomfort is usually relieved with an over-the-counter medicine similar to what you would take for a headache...and some kids take nothing at all!

FAQ #7: "Once the braces are removed, will my teeth will always stay straight?"

This is every orthodontist's dream! Unfortunately, as much as we would like to think otherwise, it will not happen without your help. The bone around your teeth constantly remodels throughout one's lifetime, so the only way to guarantee teeth stay straight is to wear a properly fitting retainer according to your orthodontist's instructions. This is the case no matter how perfect the orthodontic result. To show how seriously I believe in this, I still wear my retainers every night, and I finished orthodontic treatment a LONG time ago.

FAQ #8: "After braces, will my teeth will have scars on them?"

I would hope not. The white "scar" that sometimes is left when certain people's braces are removed is actually the first step of tooth decay. While sometimes it is reversible, many times it is not. It is caused ONLY by poor hygiene when the braces are on. If you are diligent with your home care and follow your orthodontist's instructions, the chances for this happening are ultra-low. One of my biggest disappointments is when I provide a patient with a wonderful orthodontic result, only to have their poor hygiene detract from it. This is an area that is 100% in the patient's control to prevent. No matter what you may hear or read otherwise, these "scars" have nothing to do with the type of braces used, the technique for placing braces, or length of time in treatment.

FAQ #9: "Can I wear a mouthguard for sports or play my instrument with braces?"

Absolutely on both accounts. There are several commercially available or custom mouthguards that will fit around braces. The mouthguard is so important for not only protecting the teeth and lips from injury, but also to protect the brain from concussions! Do not play ANY sports without wearing one! We will provide you with the information to select the type that is best for your needs.

It may take a few days to readjust your mouth if you play brass, but woodwinds should have no issue. Every child that I have treated with braces has continued with their musical endeavors with no problem.

FAQ #10: "I'm an adult, so what age is "too-old" to have braces?"

You are never too old! My oldest patient was 89, so I'm guessing you are probably younger than that! As long as you have the desire to improve your smile and your bite, orthodontics is appropriate to consider. Ask your child's orthodontist what options are available for adults in their office, and if you can take the smile journey along with your child!

ABOUT THE AUTHOR

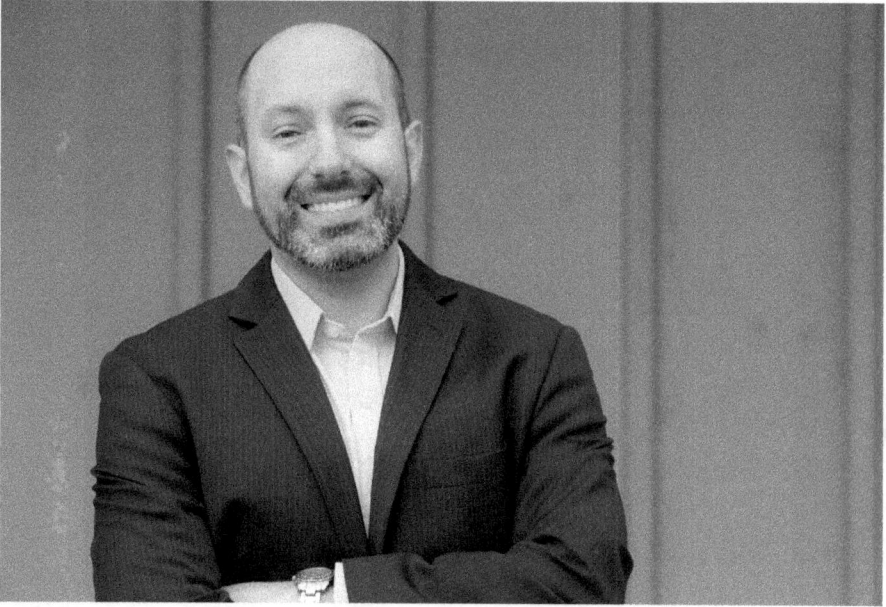

Dr. Tamburrino's Professional Details:

College: Duke University (BSE – Biomedical and Mechanical Engineering/ Materials Science)

Dental School: University of Pennsylvania School of Dental Medicine (DMD)

Orthodontic Residency: University of Pennsylvania School of Dental Medicine (Chief Resident)

Former Faculty: University of Pennsylvania School of Dental Medicine

Author: Orthodontic Treatment Design textbook, several book chapters, and scientific articles

Lecturer: Dynamic speaker at international, national, and local dental and orthodontic conferences

Co-Owner: Center for Orthodontic Excellence, with locations in Kennett Square, PA and Princeton Junction, NJ

Personal Details:

Family: Wife, two amazing sons, and two ridiculously crazy cats, Tomato and Basil

Hobbies: Golf, fitness, cooking, and model railroading

Resident: Kennett Square, PA

www.ingramcontent.com/pod-product-compliance
Lightning Source LLC
Chambersburg PA
CBHW060519280326
41933CB00014B/3033